COLORADO CLEANSE

THE
COLORADO
CLEANSE

2 Week Detox and Digestion Boot Camp

By John Douillard

LifeSpa

This book may be purchased for business or promotional use for special sales. For information, please contact us.

Internet addresses and telephone numbers given in this book were accurate at the time of publication.

Published by LifeSpa Products, LLC™ in the United States of America
First Edition – May 2010
Second Edition - October 2010
Third Edition – February 2011

Cover and Book Design by Tauna Houghton

ISBN: 978-0-615-45514-3

Dr. John Douillard's LifeSpa
6662 Gunpark Drive E, Suite 102
Boulder, CO 80301
(303) 516 – 4848
www.lifespa.com | info@lifespa.com

To Ginger

The love of my life!

ACKNOWLEDGEMENTS

I would like to say a special thanks to my amazing staff who believes so deeply in our mission here at LifeSpa. The Colorado Cleanse, which has helped so many people, couldn't have happened without all of them. In particular, I want to thank Tauna Houghton who continues to impress me with her graphic design and artistic talent. Not only did she design this book, but laid it out, did the basic editing and oversees much of the administration of the Colorado Cleanse. My thanks to Jessica Caver for her tireless administrative support, making the Colorado Cleanse happen. Thank you to Matthew Frum, our Product Manager, who has shown us all how to do much less yet accomplish much more. My deepest thanks to Briana Ybarbo who makes our front desk job look easy. Thank you to Sita Mukerji for editing the *Colorado Cleanse* book on such short notice. My gratitude to Stacy Berg whose level head is such a blessing to have watch over all of us at LifeSpa. Thank you to Nadene Moccia and Jacquelynne Stratton, our Panchakarma Therapists, who rose to the occasion when we were all overwhelmed at the response to our first Colorado Cleanse.

- John Douillard

TABLE OF CONTENTS

Success Story

~ Participating in this spring's Colorado Cleanse changed my life in profound ways. My goal was to lose a few pounds and reduce inflammation in my body. I wasn't expecting to change my eating habits but that's exactly what happened. Following the guidelines on what foods to eat and having a set regime made me realize I wasn't eating enough food. I ate sporadically, if at all, during certain times of the day. My body was in starvation mode and I didn't know it. By not eating gluten, the bloating and inflammation in my body disappeared and I lost five pounds because of it. Dairy, while I didn't eat it often, is something that contributed to my allergies and by not eating it at all, I was able to breathe better and had less sinus issues. My biggest challenge was not having sugar and coffee during the cleanse and thought it would be the first thing I would do once it ended. I'm happy to say since the Colorado Cleanse [4 months ago], I haven't had a cup of coffee and my sugar cravings are gone. I go to Starbucks regularly but now have hot water instead and skip all the cakes and desserts. If I do want something sweet, I opt for healthier options like dark or raw chocolate. Not eating gluten, dairy, common allergens, caffeine and sweeteners allowed me to be allergy free for the first time in my life. You have no idea what a gift that was in the springtime when I would normally be sneezing my head off. I sleep the best I've ever slept in my life and felt deep peace and calm throughout my body. Thank you Dr. Douillard for your wisdom and counsel during the cleanse. I'm so excited for the next one and feel more focused, stronger and healthier thanks to you! ~ A Colorado Cleanser

MEDICAL DISCLAIMER

All material provided from LifeSpa for the Colorado Cleanse is provided for informational or educational purposes only. Schedule a private consult with Dr. Douillard or with a physician regarding the applicability of any opinions or recommendations with respect to your symptoms or medical condition. The instructions and advice presented from LifeSpa for the Colorado Cleanse are in no way intended as medical advice or as a substitute for medical counseling. The information should be used in conjunction with the guidance and care of your physician. Consult your physician before beginning this program as you would any detox, weight loss or weight maintenance program. Your physician should be aware of all medical conditions that you may have as well as the medications and supplements you are taking. Those of you who are on diuretics or diabetes medication or have liver or gallbladder disease should proceed only under a doctor's supervision. As with any plan, the weight loss phases of this nutritional plan should not be used by patients on dialysis or by pregnant or nursing women.

INTRODUCTION

The Colorado Cleanse is a unique 2 week home program designed to detoxify fat soluble chemicals that store for years in the fat cells. These include heavy metals, environmental toxins, pesticides, preservatives, pollutants, parasites and plastics. Before we can successfully remove these toxins we must prepare the body's detox channels, which is the same as the digestive channels. This starts by stabilizing the blood sugar, followed with restoring normal function of the intestinal villa and the lymphatic system, which drains the gut. Then we flush and decongest the liver and gallbladder, followed by a detox of the deep tissues and fat cells.

The cleanse ends with a total reset of the digestive strength. For most of us, our ability to digest heavy or rich foods has decreased over the years. As a result of poor digestion, toxins build up and we suffer from allergies, weight gain, fatigue, sleep and mood issues – to name a few.

To see when I am leading the next guided Colorado Cleanse with live conference calls and daily emails, please visit www.lifespa.com/coloradocleanse.

Here is a general outline of the Colorado Cleanse:

PART I – General Cleansing Guidelines
During the 2 week cleanse there are specific guidelines for strengthening the digestion, de-stagnating the lymphatic system and balancing fat metabolism and blood sugar levels.

PART II – Four Day Pre-Cleanse
Balance Blood Sugar and Heal Intestinal Villa: Start by stabilizing your blood sugar and repairing the mucosa of your intestinal tract.

De-Stagnate Lymphatic System: Improve the function of your lymphatic system, which drains the gut through the GALT (Gut Associated Lymphatic Tissue) where 80% of the body's immune system is housed.

Thin the Bile and Prepare to Detox: Once the detox channels of the lymph are moving, decongest the liver and thin the bile. Adequate bile flow is critical in optimizing and maintaining the detox channels of the body.

PART III – Seven Day Main Cleanse

Reset Fat Metabolism, Flush the Liver and Detox Toxic Fat: Once the liver and bile are functioning better, cleanse the toxic chemicals that are stored in the fat cells.

Self Inquiry to Release Repetitive Mental and Emotional Patterns: Our fat cells also store old molecules of emotion, mental patterns and belief. This phase of the cleanse is a powerful time to practice self inquiry and facilitate deep transformation.

PART IV – Three Day Digestive Reset

Post Cleanse: After the cleanse, reset your upper digestive strength, which is the most common cause of digestive distress and the beginning of cellular toxicity.

Part V – Maintenance

To maximize your results I recommend that you continue the herbal protocol and the General Cleansing Guidelines for a month or longer.

Herbal Support for Cleansing

I strongly suggest that you take the recommended herbs, which will increase your benefits and make the cleanse more comfortable and effective. We sell all of these herbs at LifeSpa.com separately and in a 'Colorado Cleanse Supply Kit' (see page 161). I also make suggestions for alternative herbal strategies that are available in your health food store.

QUICK CLEANSE GUIDE

Keep this *Quick Cleanse Guide* handy so you can easily stay on track.
Please see the *Cleanse at a Glance* for a more detailed overview on page 79.

Day 1 Day 2 Day 3 Day 4	**PART II: Pre-Cleanse**<ul><li>Follow the "General Cleansing Guidelines."</li><li>Each day eat: 1-2 raw beets, 1-2 Green Smoothies, apples and drink 4 8-oz glasses of apple juice.</li><li>Eat low fat and no gluten, dairy, sugar, allergens.</li></ul>		**PART I: General Cleansing Guidelines** *(Follow during the entire cleanse.)* <ul><li>Take Before Meals: Beet Cleanse Warm Digest *or* Cool Digest Sugar Destroyer</li><li>Take After Meals: Manjistha Turmeric Plus Liver Repair Regenerate</li><li>3 meals a day, no snacks</li><li>Yoga</li><li>Breathing</li><li>Meditation</li><li>Daily Oil Massage</li><li>Exercise (with nasal breath)</li><li>Avoid: wheat, dairy, sugar, sweeteners, alcohol and drugs, coffee, oils and nuts, cold food, eggs, fish and shellfish.</li></ul>
Day 5	2 tsp ghee - am	**PART III: Main Cleanse**<ul><li>Continue with the "General Cleansing Guidelines."</li><li>Drink indicated dosage of warm ghee each morning.</li><li>Eat NONfat khichadi.</li></ul>	
Day 6	4 tsp ghee - am		
Day 7	4 tsp ghee - am		
Day 8	6 tsp ghee - am		
Day 9	8 tsp ghee - am		
Day 10	8 tsp ghee - am		
Day 11	10 tsp ghee - am 4-6 tsp castor oil - pm		
Day 12 Day 13 Day 14	**PART IV: Post-Cleanse**<ul><li>Continue the "General Cleansing Guidelines".</li><li>Follow the Digestive Strength Protocol on page 116 for Days 12-19.</li><li>Eat a Low fat diet. No gluten, dairy, sugar, allergens.</li></ul>		
Days 15-28	**PART V: Maintenance**<ul><li>Eat seasonally.</li><li>Eat wheat and dairy free, as comfortable.</li><li>Finish all herbs.</li><li>Take *Warm Digest* or *Cool Digest* as needed (such as when travelling, eating late, or eating heavy or rich foods).</li><li>Follow General Cleansing Guidelines for one more month or longer.</li></ul>		

CHAPTER 1
WHY DETOX?

The need to detoxify the body regularly has become a prerequisite for optimal health. Environmental pollutants, cancer causing chemicals, plastics, preservatives, pesticides, heavy metals and industrial waste overwhelm the body's natural detoxification pathways. Toxic cloud plumes from burning coal cover most of the United States and lace even our organic vegetables with heavy metals. Pesticides and preservatives have infiltrated their way into almost all the food consumed in America and can store in the body's fat, including the brain, for years. Industrial wastes have permeated our ground water and can enter our body by simply washing our organic veggies with tap water. Over time these stored chemicals undermine our immunity, render us susceptible to disease, infection and premature aging.

Recently the EWG, Environmental Worker's Group, reported on the amount of pesticides in our fruits and vegetables. Celery (non-organic) was found to have 67 pesticides in it even after being power washed. EWG came up with two lists:

- ❖ The Dirty Dozen: fruits and veggies with 47-67 pesticides in them.
- ❖ The Clean Fifteen: the 'clean' veggies that are usually safe if not organic.

Fortunately, the body was designed to detoxify these toxic chemicals naturally. As we age and endure higher levels of stress, our detox and digestive system weakens and a toxic world can propose a real threat. While detoxifying these chemicals regularly is critical, it is not enough. To solve this problem, we must also restore the body's natural detoxification pathways. If we only detox chemicals from fat stores into the blood stream, where do they go? They were likely stored because the body's natural detoxification system had already become inefficient. Just doing a "detox" may only relocate these chemicals from one fat cell to another. This is not only futile but dangerous as the fat located in the brain and organs are a vulnerable storage site for such toxins.

The Colorado Cleanse is designed to reset natural detoxification pathways so the body can protect itself from a toxic world.

Household Toxin Report

These 5 Dangerous Household Toxins are in Every Room!

These toxins are linked to sexual, nervous system and behavioral problems like Attention Deficit Syndrome as well as many cancers. These chemicals find their way into breast milk in infants and fetuses which makes their impact far greater than previously believed according to CNN and the Environmental Workers Group.[1,2]

Toxin #1: BPA's Bisphenols
- ❖ Plastics found in water bottles, baby bottles, cans and other plastic products. If the plastic bottle has a recycle number of 7 it is toxic.
- ❖ Solution: Drink from stainless steel containers and use BPA-free tupperware to store food.

Toxin #2: Phthalates
- ❖ These fragrances are not required to be listed in the ingredients of personal care products like creams, shampoos and lotions. They are also hormonal disruptors that store in the body for years.
- ❖ Solution: Use only 100% preservative free products, such as our completely natural skin care line. www.lifespa.com/skincare.

Toxin #3: Perfluorooctanic acid PFOAs.
- ❖ These are found in Teflon and water resistant clothing.
- ❖ Solution: Use cast iron or stainless steel pots and natural fiber clothing.

Toxin #4: Formaldehyde
- ❖ Found in pressed wood and glues - a known carcinogen.
- ❖ Solution: Buy only whole wood furniture and avoid particle board.

Toxin #5: Polybrominated diphenyl ethers
- ❖ These are flame retardants and are everywhere: in clothes, bedding, carports, TVs, electronics, etc. They end up in the dust we breathe and make their way into children, infants and fetuses. They damage the liver and kidney and - like the rest - affect the brain function and behavior.
- ❖ Solution: Dust and vacuum regularly. Specifically around and in the back of electronics.

These *5 Most Toxic Household Chemicals* are found in almost every room in most homes:

- storage containers
- food wrap
- cans
- cookware
- appliances
- carpets
- shower curtains
- clothes
- personal care products
- fragrances
- furniture
- televisions
- electronics
- bedding
- mattresses
- dust

The Dirty Dozen

While the FDA tells us that all fruits and veggies have safe and harmless levels of pesticides, The President's Cancer Panel recommends consumers eat produce without pesticides to reduce the risk of cancer and disease.

While long term studies have not been completed, some research links pesticides with cancer, ADD, nervous system and immune disorders.

The Dirty Dozen were power-washed before testing. Washing is important to remove bacteria but obviously has little effect on removing pesticides. If you are going to buy any of the fruits or veggies listed in The Dirty Dozen we highly recommend buying only organic.

The Dirty Dozen
Foods to always buy organic.

Celery
Peaches
Strawberries
Apples
Blueberries
Nectarines
Sweet Bell Peppers
Spinach, Kale, Collard Greens
Cherries
Potatoes
Grapes
Lettuce

Soft-skinned fruits and vegetables are typically the most toxic when not organic.

The Clean Fifteen

To ensure that you and your family are safe and healthy, eat organic whenever possible. The Clean Fifteen are fruits and vegetables that are considered safe by the EWG to eat even when not organic.

Nature's Natural Detox

Every spring and fall certain foods are harvested that naturally provoke a cleansing response in the body. Sadly, most of us eat the same foods 365 days of the year and miss out on this seasonal detoxification. Today - in a world that has become more toxic than ever - seasonal detoxification is required.

After a long winter of heavy, insulating, warming and holiday foods, the intestinal tract can become boggy and congested in the spring. The hair-like villi become compromised at the end of winter and early spring because of these heavy foods. These villi drain fat soluble toxins and nutrition off the gut wall into the lymph and blood stream. Spring is a wet, rainy and muddy time of year that can add to the congestion of the intestinal tract, further bogging down the villi and stagnating the lymph drainage around the gut where 80% of the body's immune system lives.

In the fall, after a long hot summer, similar imbalances occur in the digestive system. Because summer heat tends to dry the mucus membranes in the gut, they compensate by reactively producing excessive mucus which bogs down the villi and congests the lymph. The lymphatic system pulls toxins off of the intestinal lining and neutralizes them with white blood cells. Lymph vessels act as drains for the entire body. Without a lymphatic system, we wouldn't have an

> **The Clean Fifteen**
> *These foods are considered safe even when not organic.*
>
> Onions
> Avocados
> Sweet Corn
> Pineapples
> Mango
> Sweet Peas
> Asparagus
> Kiwi
> Cabbage
> Eggplant
> Cantaloupe
> Watermelon
> Grapefruit
> Sweet Onions
> Sweet Potatoes

immune system and would be dead in 14 hours. Therefore, optimal lymphatic flow is essential. Let's look at how nature cares for this precious system.

Spring and fall harvested roots cleanse and pull toxic mucus off the gut wall and villi. Roots like dandelion, turmeric, goldenseal, oregon grape, ginger, fenugreek, phyllanthus and picorhiza are great intestinal villi mucus pullers. At LifeSpa I use two formulas for this: *Liver Repair* and *Turmeric Plus*.

In the fall, seasonal fruits like apples and pomegranates act as detoxifiers for the gut wall and villi. These and other fall harvested fruits are great lymph movers and help to de-stagnate the lymphatic system, which commonly becomes congested.

In the spring, shortly after the roots are harvested, the chlorophyll rich sprouts surface and the valleys turn fluorescent green. These spring greens provide the fertilizer to grow good bacteria on the intestinal villi. These good bacteria that line all the villi control the efficiency of digestion, assimilation and detoxification. Every spring and fall after the bitter roots remove excess mucus congestion in the gut, the greens – if eaten in abundance - will seed the villi with essential good bacteria and flush the lymphatic system.

Once the villi have been cleansed with roots and then fertilized with greens each spring and fall, nature moves to cleanse the lymph that surrounds the outside of the gut wall. In the spring this is done with leafy greens, berries and cherries which are harvested towards the end of season. In the fall the lymph is cleansed by more leafy greens, apples, pomegranates, and other seasonal fruit, as well as by beets, cranberries and assorted wild berries that are also fall harvested. The main herbs that I use for de-stagnating the lymphatic system are **Manjistha,** *Turmeric Plus* and **Red Root**.

Each spring and fall, if these foods are eaten in abundance, a natural detoxification will result. Many of us however, like myself, never seem to get around to eating enough of these seasonal roots, greens, fruits and berries. So I detoxify twice a year with herbs and a cleanse to make sure I am not accumulating dangerous toxins in my lymph, liver and fat. Please don't miss nature's opportunity to detoxify each spring and fall.

"I Can't Eat Fat!"

Now, let's say you have not been cleansing twice a year and your body is toxic. How does the body deal with this? Unfortunately, after the lymph and villi become congested - which is extremely common - the toxins default back to the liver. The liver, which is usually overwhelmed, will often redirect these toxins back into the blood to be stored in fats cells somewhere in the body or the brain. Along the way, liver function and bile flow slow down and it becomes more challenging for the body to metabolize fats. This is a primary reason for high cholesterol, weight gain and an inability to digest fatty or greasy foods. Without the ability to digest fats well, we also lose the ability to make energy last, sleep through the night, neutralize the degenerative chemistry of stress and detox dangerous cancer causing chemicals and molecules of emotion.

Fat metabolism helps to stabilize blood sugar and create a calm mood in addition to balancing healthy weight. Many people attempt to fix this problem by eating small, frequent meals that are easier to digest but unfortunately do not address the cause. We must heal the intestinal villa and restore normal lymphatic flow.

"I Can't Eat Wheat or Dairy"

When liver function and bile flow decrease, the bile is not able to buffer stomach acids when they leave the stomach and enter the small intestine, which can cause heart burn and indigestion. The stomach responds by turning down its fire, resulting in the inability to break down hard-to-digest proteins like gluten in wheat and casein in dairy.

Without a strong digestive system, tough cancer causing toxins and parasites now pass right on through the stomach and become irritants to the intestinal mucosa. As the intestinal mucus membranes inflame, the villi become further compromised and the lymph becomes more stagnant.

This cycle continues until we repair these digestive and detox pathways and then detoxify the cancer-causing fat soluble toxins that hide deep in our fatty tissue. As we age, these chemicals often rear their ugly heads as provoking agents for disease and illness.

This is why here at LifeSpa we are so dedicated to cleansing - but only if it is a program that also restores optimal digestive and detox pathways so that the body can naturally protect itself from a toxic environment in the future.

Welcome to the Colorado Cleanse.

References
1. EWG, Environmental Worker's Group
2. CNN: "Toxic America" May 31, 2010

Success Story
~ My bladder pain went away completely. I started having bowel movements again. My insulin requirements decreased to half. My depression which was severe, went to moderate/minimal. I stopped all estrogen and other hormones, without any noticeable effect. (In the past, even one night was impossible.) I also stopped all pancreatic enzymes, iron and other supplements, which I had felt were keeping me afloat. I had no problem this week being without any of those.

CHAPTER 2
RELEASE MENTAL AND EMOTIONAL STRESS

Recently, fascinating research that found 95% of the body's serotonin in the intestinal wall and only 5% in the brain where we typically think serotonin is stored and manufactured.[1]

Clinically this is incredibly relevant because I track the cause of disease the best I can in my practice and almost always find myself looking down the barrel of emotional patterns of behavior that were created many years ago in order to feel safe as the cause of disease. These emotional strains are processed through the intestinal wall, and then delivered to the brain then the body as a stress response.

The problem is that while the intestines are the processing center of stress, the digestive fire goes out, the intestinal wall inflames, assimilation and detoxification channels break down and we start avoiding the foods that we have a hard time digesting and instead just label them "bad foods".

What is amazing is that Ayurvedic doctors knew 5000 years ago that mental and emotional stress caused disease and that 80% of disease was treated through the digestive system. They knew that the intestines were the "second brain" and that emotional stress would cause digestive imbalances that would in turn impact every cell in the body.

These mental and emotional stressors produce neurotransmitters referred to as molecules of emotion that, according to Ayurveda, store in fat cells and must be released to make needed transformational changes that unlock the digestive imbalances and the disease process. This is just one of the reasons why is it so crucial to become a good fat burner.

In one recent study, 14 of the major fat soluble cancer causing toxic chemicals that store in the body's fat cells were detoxified during Pancahakarma - an Ayurvedic Detox Retreat we offer at the LifeSpa in Boulder, Colorado. After this seven day cleanse, much of which the Colorado Cleanse is modeled after, the body continued to detoxify these cancer causing chemicals for 3 months.[2]

The molecules of emotion or what Ayurveda calls "Mental Toxins" are also fat soluble and store in the muscle and fat cells all over the body. When under stress, recurring neurotransmitters are released which carry the emotional message and trigger repetitive and reactive patterns of behavior that make us do the same dumb stuff again and again.

The body must be able to burn fat well to release the toxic chemicals and molecules of emotion from the fat cells in order to open the door to changing these old emotional patterns. During the Colorado Cleanse the body is forced to release toxic and emotional fat stores, which gives you, the cleanser, the opportunity to transform old emotional patterns that lock the body and mind in imbalanced behavior that is typically undesirable.

During the Main Cleanse, I offer a series of Self Inquiry exercises that will ensure the transformation of old emotions once they are released from the deep fat stores in the body during the cleanse.

The Colorado Cleanse is designed to remove the density of the physical body in order for us to have the clarity to see and transform the mental and emotional patterns that have driven the body into imbalance and pain. Once the body starts cleansing at this deep level, Self Inquiry is a critical tool to fully detoxify and transform the body, mind and spirit.

During Panchakarma, which includes the components of the Colorado Cleanse, numerous studies document the powerful transformational process for those who don't digest well, have lost the ability to detox on their own and have deep underlying emotional patterns of behavior that have locked in these mental, physical and emotional imbalances.

Recent research has documented these benefits:

- ❖ Decreases cholesterol, by lowering toxic lipid peroxide levels.[4]
- ❖ Decrease the rate of platelet clumping and thus lymphatic congestion.[5]
- ❖ Decreases 14 major toxic and cancer causing chemicals from body tissues including heavy metals, pesticides and other hazardous environmental chemicals.[2]
- ❖ Significantly raised the good HDL cholesterols.[6]
- ❖ Lowered diastolic blood pressure.[5]
- ❖ Reduced free radicals which are the leading cause of all disease, cancer and death.[4]
- ❖ Significant reductions in bodily complaints, irritability, bodily strain, and psychological inhibition, as well as greater emotional stability. [4]
- ❖ Decreased anxiety, aging and reduced doctors visits.[6]

References

1. Gershon MD. 5-HT (Serotonin) physiology and related drugs. Curr Opin Gastroenterol 2000; 16: 113–20.DO
2. Herron, Fagan. Alternative Therapies in Health and Medicine, September/October 2002. Panchakarma therapy greatly reduces the levels of 14 important 'lipophilic' (i.e. fat-soluble) toxic and carcinogenic chemicals in the body.
3. Schneider RH, Cavanaugh KL, Kasture HS, Rothenberg S, Averbach R, Robinson D, Wallace RK. Health promotion with a traditional system of natural health care: Maharishi Ayur-Veda. Journal of Social Behavior and Personality, 1990, 5(3): 1-27.
4. Nidich SI, Smith DE, Sands D, Sharma H, Nidich RJ, Barnes V, Jossang S. Effect of Maharishi Ayur-Ved Panchakarma purification program on speed of processing ability. Maharishi International University, Fairfield, Iowa, USA.
5. Sharma HM, Nidich SI, Sands D, Smith DE. Improvement in cardiovascular risk factors through Panchakarma purification procedures. Journal of Research and Education in Indian Medicine, 1993, XII: 4, 2-13.
6. Waldschutz R. Veranderungen physiologischer und psychischer Parameter durch eine ayurvedische Reinigungskur. Erfahrungsheilkunde - Acta Medica Empirica, 1988, 11: 720-729.

CHAPTER 3
STOP EATING DAIRY UNTIL YOU READ THIS!

Dairy, much like gluten, has been deemed by many to be a "bad food". Some studies have linked dairy products to just about everything - from allergies to obesity, fatigue, mood, instability and more.

Other studies promote compelling research that link dairy to numerous health benefits and tout it as an essential food for optimal health.

With both camps citing conflicting studies the truth about dairy is confusing, to say the least.

Dairy Is Not Required
It should be clear that there are many cultures around the world that do not eat dairy products. Most of preindustrial Africa and Asia, with the exception of India and Hindu cultures, rarely consumed milk. That being said, Northern European cultures have been healthily eating dairy for thousands of years.

You Don't Have to Eat Dairy to Be Healthy
Even though dairy has been healthily ingested and even used as medicine for thousands of years, it is not required to eat dairy products in order to be healthy. Raw milk, as nature intended, is a very good source of fat soluble vitamins and protein that Northern Europeans, Indians (India) and many other cultures used. Below I describe how traditional cultures solved many of today's dairy problems thousands of years ago with Ayurvedic principles.

Lactose Intolerance Isn't New
After the age of four many people, and up to 90% of blacks and Asians, stop making the enzyme lactase which makes them potentially lactose intolerant.[1] Milk sugar is called lactose and needs the enzyme lactase to be digested. DNA evidence extracted from Neolithic skeletons indicates that in 5500 BC, people in Northern Europe were also lactose intolerant.[2] Earthenware vessels found in

England and dated to 4500 BC contain milk byproducts, indicating milk was used in some form, although perhaps not drunk directly. [3]

Symptoms of Lactose Intolerance
The signs and symptoms of lactose intolerance usually begin 30 minutes after eating or drinking foods that contain lactose.

Common signs and symptoms include:
- nausea
- sinus congestion
- abdominal cramps
- bloating
- gas
- diarrhea

Lactose Intolerant People Can Eat Some Specific Types of Dairy
In cheese, and particularly cottage cheese, the lactose is converted to lactic acid which is easy digest.

Folks with lactose intolerance should be able to eat cheese. [4]

Cream, butter and yogurt have very small amounts of lactose and are usually okay.

Skim milk still has lactose, so it is not a choice for lactose intolerant folks.

Isn't Dairy a Needed Source of Calcium for Building Bones? No!
While calcium, vitamins and other minerals are abundant in certain types of milk, calcium is way more abundant in leafy green veggies. There are many non dairy cultures that have incredible bone density without consuming milk products. [5]

Excellent Sources of Calcium:
- Fresh, dark-green vegetables like spinach, kale, turnips, collard greens

- ❖ Legumes
- ❖ Sesame seeds and almonds
- ❖ Wild salmon and sardines
- ❖ Rhubarb
- ❖ Okra

Vitamin D$_3$ Is More Important For Building Strong Bones Than Calcium

The biggest factor regarding calcium absorption is getting adequate amounts of Vitamin D$_3$, which we primarily absorb from the sun or supplementation.

In the cream portion of milk there is a good supply of Vitamin D$_3$, along with the other essential fat soluble vitamins A, E and K. Unfortunately these vitamins are broken down in the pasteurization and homogenization process. As a result, milk is fortified with synthetic Vitamin A, D2 (not Vitamin D$_3$) and calcium. More importantly, 78% of Americans are Vitamin D$_3$ Deficient - yet Vitamin D$_3$ is required to carry the dietary calcium out of the gut and into the bloodstream.

If You Want Strong Bones Get Your Vitamin D$_3$

It is the chronic deficiency of Vitamin D$_3$ that causes most calcium deficiencies and osteoporosis.

While raw milk is a better source of fat soluble vitamins and calcium than conventionally pasteurized milk, it still does not deliver enough Vitamin D$_3$ to benefit from the numerous health advantages of Vitamin D$_3$ optimization. Vitamin D$_3$ supplementation in the winter and regular midday sun exposure in the summer is strongly recommended for optimal health and strong bones. Learn more at www.lifespa.com/VitaminD.

Should I Just Drink Skim Milk To Be Safe? No!

Skim milk is made from skimming off the cream that normally rises to the surface, which makes it nonfat and thus completely lacking in essential fat soluble Vitamins A, D$_3$, E and K. Yet skim milk still has the proteins and lactose that can cause allergies, lactose intolerance and indigestion.

Milk is 80% casein protein and 20% whey protein. The proteins in milk are the most common culprit when it comes to indigestion and allergies. Casein, in particular, is very hard to digest. Mother's milk has four times the amount of easy to digest whey protein and one-half the amount of hard to digest casein protein than cow's milk. So it seems we were never meant to digest lots of casein. Since both of these proteins are water soluble, they remain in the skim milk, making it a richer source of protein - but much more difficult to digest.

It is also common to think that skim milk is better than whole milk for lactose intolerance, but the lactose also remains in the skim non fat milk - again making it much harder to digest.

Mother's milk also has five times the linoleic acid than cow's milk, which is a fat critical for building the nervous system and intelligence. [6] Skimming milk takes the small amount of linoleic acid out of the milk, along with the needed fats, so it will lack the support whole milk provides for the nervous system.

Skim Milk Is Hard to Digest and Lacks Nutrients
Skimming the fat off milk creates a higher protein, higher mineral beverage that is more difficult to digest. The fats in milk – except skim milk - build and balance the nervous system and act as carriers to deliver the calcium and fat soluble Vitamins A, D3,E and K directly into the cells.

Skim milk though, is a less toxic option..... See why below!

If You Can't Get Raw Dairy Choose Vat Pasteurized Products
This is a hotly debated topic and may be the most confusing. Pasteurization is a process that heats milk in order to kill food borne bacteria, microbes and pathogens. While pasteurization has saved countless lives when dairy farms were less than sanitary - today many take issue with this process.

By killing the bad bacteria, the good bacteria are also killed, along with the enzymes so desperately needed to break down the hard to digest proteins and fats and deliver the vitamins and minerals. Raw milk advocates, such as the

Weston Price Foundation, link pasteurization to high cholesterol, atherosclerosis, sinus congestion and the litany of health concerns blamed on dairy products.

There are 3 kinds of pasteurization that you might see written on a label:

Vat Pasteurized
BEST Commercial Choice
Heats milk to 135 degrees for 20 minutes.
Shelf life 7-10 days. It's still alive!
Preserves good bacteria and many enzymes.

Pasteurized
TRY TO AVOID
Traditional process: Heats milk to 160 degrees for 15-20 seconds.
Shelf life 2-3 weeks.
Preserves some good bacteria.

Ultra Pasteurized
AVOID
Heats milk to 275 degrees for a couple of seconds.
Shelf life 2-3 months.
Kills everything.

Vat Pasteurization is becoming a more popular option. It provides a guaranteed bacteria free product while preserving many of the enzymes and good bacteria because the heat is relatively low.

Organic Valley just released a whole milk product that is vat pasteurized and non-homogenized. Kalona Farms in Iowa, which also distributes nationally, offers a variety of vat pasteurized non-homogenized products.

Avoid Pasteurization and Always Boil Your Milk
According to Ayurveda, heating the milk slowly to just when it starts to boil will kill the bacteria and pathogens but leave the good bacteria and the enzymes.

Heating the milk too fast at high temperatures for just a second or two during conventional "Flash" pasteurization will of course kill all the bacteria but also partially breaks down the hard to digest protein chains, leaving them extremely difficult to digest. [7]

Bringing already pasteurized milk to a boil will finish the job of breaking down the proteins and make them easier to digest. If you buy pasteurized milk, bring it slowly to a boil, let it cool and drink... Avoid Ultra Pasteurization. Look for Vat Pasteurized – or better yet, choose raw products.

For best digestibility bring them to a boil as well.

Always Buy Organic Dairy Products
One of the problems with non organic dairy is that the chemicals, hormones and toxins in our world are generally fat soluble. Milk is high on the food chain and toxins are therefore passed through the feed into the milk and carried in the fatty portion of the milk. The only way to avoid the overwhelming amounts of antibiotics, growth hormones and pesticides in milk is to buy organic where these fat soluble chemicals are not present.

Choose Organic (or Skim Milk if there is no other option)
If you have to drink non organic milk, choose skim milk. Yes, though it is harder to digest it is basically devoid of fat and will not carry the hormones, antibiotics and pesticides that whole or low fat milk would. Skim Milk is the only relatively safe non organic option.

Homogenization Causes Most Dairy Intolerance
From the Ayurvedic perspective and that of many researchers, the homogenization process renders the fat in milk indigestible. The fat (cream) molecules are squeezed through a small filter in order to make them homogenous or the same. This homogenous fat is a foreign molecule to the body. Often this molecule will pass undigested through weakened small intestinal linings, and makes foreign sludge in the lymph and blood stream which sticks to channel walls, creates plaque and allergic responses. [8]

Some researchers believe this process allows a toxic enzyme called xanthine oxidase to enter into the blood stream and cause damage to the arterial wall. This arterial free radical damage causes scar tissue to form. Cholesterol accumulates on the scars and clogs the arteries. [9]

Choose Organic Whipping Cream When Raw Products are Not Available
Since almost all commercial milk is homogenized there are only a few strategies to avoid homogenized dairy products. Skim milk is homogenized. Residual amounts of fat remain after the skimming process that is then homogenized.

The Best Choice is Organic Raw Milk
The only other non-homogenized milk product is heavy whipping cream. The cream is skimmed off and never homogenized. Because whipping cream will not whip when ultra pasteurized, all whipping cream is always pasteurized at lower temperatures, which also spares enzymes and good bacteria. Choose organic because the fat in cream is a carrier for fat soluble toxins.

Organic Valley sells Organic Whipping Cream that is non-homogenized and vat pasteurized. This is the best of both worlds. You can add water to dilute the cream to the desired consistency. Cream is also where the easy to digest constituents are found. It is where the linoleic acid, Vitamins A,D,E and K, minerals and other healthy fats are found. Cream is much easier to digest because it is almost devoid of lactose and hard to digest proteins.

Dilute Whipping Cream with Water for Your Own Health Promoting Milk
Traditionally, milk was never consumed in big glasses like in the west. Because milk is high in hard to digest proteins and lactose, it was traditionally allowed to separate from the cream. The cream was eaten in the raw form and saved for cooking, and the skim milk was made into cheese or yogurt, which made the proteins and lactose easier to digest. The cream was diluted with water for almost all cooking purposes when milk was called for. Cream provided the fats, vitamins and some minerals directly and cheese provided a high protein, high mineral product that was easy to digest.

Solution: Organic whipping cream and organic cottage cheese are available almost everywhere these days. What a simple solution to such a complicated problem!

Raw Organic Milk Is Your Best Choice
If you choose to drink milk on a regular basis, the best choice is Raw Organic Milk. I still suggest that you bring it to a boil before drinking it and that you always drink it warm or at room temperature, never cold. Then you will have an easy to digest, non congesting and extremely nutritious beverage.

Unfortunately it is difficult to get raw milk. It is mostly sold through local farm shares. Go to RealMilk.com to find a farm share in your area.

The Real Question is "Why Are You Allergic to Dairy?"
As I have written and lectured about for many years, dairy is a hard to digest food. That is why Ayurvedic medicine suggested separating the cream, which is easy to digest, from the protein rich skim, which is difficult to digest.

While eating the healthiest form of dairy makes total sense, just changing the diet is never enough. If you have difficulty digesting something that is hard to digest, evaluate the strength and integrity of the digestive process. One of the main points of the Colorado Cleanse is the reset of original digestive strength so that hard to digest foods – that many folks avoid – can be eaten once again. If you don't digest dairy well you do not have to eat it - just be sure it is not a sign of a weakened digestive system... If so, let's fix it!

Related Health Reports:
- ❖ *Poor Digestion Linked to Cancer* (www.lifespa.com/constipation)
- ❖ *Surprising Symptoms Linked to Poor Digestion* (www.lifespa.com/DigestiveHealth)
- ❖ *The Miracle of Lymph* (www.lifespa.com/Lymph)
- ❖ *Look and Feel Vibrant in 3 Steps* - learn how to care for your 'inner skin', which is an important part of your digestion (www.lifespa.com/Skin)

❖ *Top 10 Proven Weight Loss Tips* - this Health Report is really about having excellent digestion (www.lifespa.com/Top10)
❖ *The Hidden Dangers of Enzymes!* (www.lifespa.com/Enzymes)

References
1. J. Bayless, Lactose and Milk Intolerance: Clinical Impressions, N Engl J Med, 292 (1975)
2. Early man "couldn't stomach milk, 27 February 2007, news.bbc.co.uk. Retrieved on 21 July 2009.
3. Stone Age Man Drank Milk". London: Independent.co.uk. 2003-01-28. www.independent.co.uk/news/science/stone-age-man-drank-milk-scientists-find-605237.html. Retrieved 2010-08-28.
4. McDougall. The McDougall Plan, New Century Books p. 50
5. Walker, Osteoporosis and Calcium Deficiency, Am J Clin Nutr 16, 1965
6. M. Crawford, Essential Fatty Acids Requirements in Infancy, Am J Clin Nutr 31 (1978)
7. Ballentine, Diet and Nutrition. Honesdale, Himalayan Institute.. 1978, p.129 Oster, K., 8. Oster, J., and Ross, D. "Immune Response to Bovine Xanthine Oxidase in Atherosclerotic Patients." American Laboratory, August, 1974, 41-47
8. Oster, K., and Ross, D. "The Presence of Ectopic Xanthine Oxidase in Atherosclerotic Plaques and Myocardial Tissues." Proceedings of the Society for Experimental Biology and Medicine, 1973.

Success Story
~ I am obese and 3 years ago I started on a journey to shed my excess weight. I became stuck on a plateau and despite all of my efforts I wound up regaining some of the weight. This went on for nearly 2 years (seriously) until I did the Spring 2010 Colorado Cleanse and I have lost about 60 pounds total since the May cleanse. I truly believe that detoxing my fat cells and cleaning and healing my GI tract has truly fundamentally changed how my body works. I am thrilled!

CHAPTER 4
SECRETS TO ENJOYING GLUTEN AGAIN

During the last twenty years or so, gluten has been accused of causing allergies, chronic fatigue, insomnia, auto-immune conditions, attention deficit disorder, asthma, memory loss, focus issues, headaches, rashes, joint pain, digestive issues, malaise, anxiety, depression, cravings and exhaustion - to name a few. In America we are innocent until proven guilty and I think gluten has been convicted without a fair trial. Giving gluten a life sentence with only symptomatic evidence just isn't right! Let's dig in here and find out the truth about gluten.

10,000 Years of Gluten
Gluten is a protein that has been eaten for 10,000 years all around the world and still is to this day. It is most commonly found in wheat but also found in many other grains.

Undigested Gluten is the Problem –
Not Gluten Itself
There are good studies that have shown that the undigested protein molecule of gluten can cause Leaky Gut Syndrome. This is a syndrome where the villi of the small intestine become damaged and begin to separate, which causes the spaces in the semi-permeable membrane of the small intestines to break down. Undigested proteins, pathogens and fat soluble toxins can sneak into the blood and lymph before they are neutralized by the digestive system. In two of my health reports *The Miracle of the Lymph* and *Look and Feel Vibrant in 3 Steps*, I explained that 80% of the body's immune response is located in the gut. When these villi get beaten up by undigested

Gluten-Rich Grains

Barley
Bulgar
Couscous
Durum
Einkorn
Kamut
Malt
Semolina
Spelt
Triticale
Rye
Wheat
Wheat bran
Wheat germ
Wheat starch
Oats – are *usually OK, but look for a brand that says 'not contaminated with wheat'*

gluten you can begin to see why a host of symptoms arise and why gluten has been given a life sentence.

>>> Learn More - Free Health Report and Videos:
  ❖ *The Miracle of Lymph*: www.lifespa.com/lymph
  ❖ *Look and Feel Vibrant in 3 Steps*: www.lifespa.com/skin

Weak Digestive Fire Can't Cook Gluten

Gluten is a very hard to digest protein that requires a specifically strong acid in the stomach to process it. Without optimal digestive fire, gluten will not be broken down in the stomach. If gluten passes through the stomach undigested, it will - if eaten in excess - cause irritation to the intestinal villi.

Though it is common for the strength of the stomach acids and the overall digestive strength to weaken over time, it is not due to the aging process. This is a very reversible condition at any age. If we don't reset the digestive strength, a host of symptoms such as toxicity, food allergies, gluten intolerance and deficiencies will ensue.

As it turns out, gluten is not particularly bad. It is simply a harder protein to break down that can wreak havoc on the gut wall if our digestion has become too weak to digest it. We are told, "Stop eating wheat and all your problems go away."

Well some of them do disappear - for a while - until the problems start to return again. Then we take other hard to digest foods off the diet - such as dairy, corn, nuts, soy, fish and so on - until eating becomes a very challenging venture.

Secrets to Enjoying Gluten Again

First we must diagnose why the stomach acids have been turned off in the first place and why we can no longer digest richer or heavier foods. The main causes are dehydration, lymph congestion, thick bile, congested liver, inflamed intestinal villi and stress, all of which we address in the Colorado Cleanse. For more information on this topic check out these Health Reports:

❖ *Surprising Symptoms of Poor Digestion* (www.lifespa.com/digestivehealth).
❖ *Top 10 Weight Loss Tips*, which is really about improving digestion. (www.lifespa.com/top10)
❖ *The Miracle of Lymph* (www.lifespa.com/lymph)

Start Your Engines

Usually the stomach acids have been turned off for a reason and we must identify that first. Often, with good habits, the body balances itself and all that is needed is to turn the digestive fire back on. For this I use a technique called The Digestive Strength Protocol, which you will do during the Post Cleanse (on page 116).

Gluten Isn't Meant to Be Eaten Every Day of the Year

The other secret about gluten and wheat is that it was never meant to be eaten three times a day, every day of the year. This overwhelming amount of gluten, along with increasing stress, will bog down the digestive process and begin to let the gluten through the stomach without being properly broken down.

Wheat and most other glutinous grains are harvested in the fall and thus eaten in the winter. This heavy, warm, wet protein rich grain is the perfect antidote for the coldness and dryness of winter. Interestingly, according to Ayurveda, our digestive strength and fire is strongest in the winter. We can digest the hard to digest foods in the season they are harvested. In the spring, which is a damp, heavy, wet time of year, this grain is not available if you are eating based on natural harvesting cycles.

A Gluten Free Spring

After a long winter of eating heavy, insulating foods rich in proteins and fat, nature changes the harvest and gives us a fat free and gluten free harvest each spring. It takes about 6-8 weeks without gluten to heal and repair the villi and nature has designed this digestive rest to happen each spring:

❖ Leafy greens fertilize the villi with new healthy bacteria.
❖ Bitter roots that are harvested each spring, like dandelion and turmeric, cleanse the villi of excessive mucus.

❖ The berries and cherries of late spring de-stagnate the Gut Associated Lymphatic Tissue that resides just on the outer wall in the intestinal tract.
❖ Follow my Spring Tips and Grocery List at www.lifespa.com/grocery.
❖ Grain alternatives include: amaranth, quinoa, millet, rice, potatoes, or rice cakes.

Ancient Techniques to Help Digest Gluten

I am always amazed at how traditional cultures developed successful techniques to help them enjoy the tastes and benefits of wheat and gluten. Sourdough bread is one of them. The culture of the sourdough goes through a fermentation process that breaks down the gluten protein and renders it much easier to digest. So look for a good quality sourdough bread and toast it for added digestibility.

One other technique to help the stomach win the battle of breaking down the gluten protein is to soak your grains overnight. This softens the grain and activates enzymes within the grain that begin to break down and release this protein.

Here are some ideas:

Soak oats (or other cereal grains) overnight before cooking them for breakfast

Soak grains like barley and bulgar before turning them into a delicious soup, casserole or stew

Conclusion: Eat Smart

If you abuse gluten, over eat it and let your digestive fires weaken, it will have its way with you. With strong digestion, which we can rekindle, and respect of natural harvest cycles, most of us can enjoy the taste and benefits of wheat for many more years to come.

CHAPTER 5
BE FIT IN 12 MINUTES A DAY

I am often asked, "What is the best exercise?," "Why don't I lose weight when I exercise?, "Whenever I start an exercise program I get injured – how can I avoid this?"

During appropriate exercise, fat replaces sugar as your main fuel supply and you naturally lose weight, detoxify, boost energy, stabilize mood and - oh yes - get really fit!

New research shows how this can be done in as little as 12 minutes a day![1,2,4] This is a simple and doable amount of exercise during the Colorado Cleanse.

How I Became a Better Athlete

In 1981, I went to hear my first lecture on Ayurveda, India's 5000 year old natural system of medicine. At the time I was training for an Ironman Triathlon. I was exhausted, getting dizzy in classes and beginning to wonder if I was doing too much. So I asked this Ayurvedic doctor, "I am training for a triathlon where you swim 2.4 miles, bike 112 miles and run 26 miles. Do you think this is healthy according to your system?"

He responded, "Why are you doing it?"

I responded, wimpishly, after an awkward moment of realizing I had no idea why I was doing it, " Because I think I can do it."

He responded, "Do you meditate?" (*Suggesting that if I meditated you wouldn't attempt such a foolish thing.*)

I proudly responded, "Yes I do meditate"

He said, "Do you sleep when you meditate?"

I said proudly. "Absolutely, I fall into the deepest sleep imaginable - every time!"

He responded, "Sleep and meditation are different. When you meditate you should not sleep. Sleeping during meditation means you are exhausted and probably exercising too much".

So I suggested, "If I can meditate without falling asleep, then the amount of exercise I am doing is OK, correct?"

He said, "Correct."

I Had My Marching Orders

I started exercising less and meditating more with hopes to not fall asleep. To my surprise, this was really hard. I realized I was quite exhausted because I slept every time I tried to meditate. Runs were shortened from hours to 15 minutes where I would sprint most of the way with periods of recovery. Bike rides were shortened to 15-20 minute sprints and recoveries from Redondo to Manhattan Beach where I would commute a couple of times a day.

At that time I was competing in a couple of triathlons a month but was never able to compete on the elite level I knew I was capable of. Training harder or longer wasn't working. I reached a point where I just wasn't improving.

Do Less, Accomplish More

Within a couple months of following my new training regime of working out less and meditating more – basically getting more rest and exercising more efficiently - I started placing in the top ten in some of my races. Many of my friends thought I was doing steroids, which I wasn't. It was clear this was really working, to the point where I was able to compete in a couple of pro races and still do quite well.

This experience of doing less and accomplishing more was so incredible to me that I passionately wanted to know more about Ayurveda. I went to India where I did years of study and wrote my first book, *Body, Mind and Sport* which reported on our research of what were then unorthodox training techniques. (*The above story is taken from the last chapter in Body, Mind and Sport called "Jet Fuel" where I discussed in more detail my personal success with these techniques*).

Fast Forward Thirty Years

This summer I competed in my first triathlon in 26 years! The best part is that I did it with my 20, 18 and 14 year old kids!!! It was a dream come true. With six kids and a busy life, my old training techniques of shorter and more efficient workouts combining cycles of sprints and rest paid great dividends, placing me first in my age group.

After years of training theories that include 45 minutes on the treadmill or an hour at the gym, the majority of folks are still not exercising regularly. Recently, the understanding of how to get the most out of your exercise has dramatically shifted. Interestingly, these new studies closely resemble what I stumbled upon almost 30 years ago.

Chasing the Rabbit

Historically, we would exercise as a way of survival. Hunting a rabbit wouldn't require 45 minutes in your heart rate training zone three times a week. It would require multiple sprints that would last about a minute, followed by periods of rest while you wait for the rabbit to show again. A natural fitness level was achieved after a handful of attempts sprinting after the rabbit followed by subsequent periods of rest and recovery.

These discussions of shorter workouts with sprints seem to be the topic of many magazine articles today. Twenty five years ago, Dr. Irv Dardik introduced a theory called "heart rate variability training" which I love. Heart rate variability means training your heart rate to be able to go really high in a sprint and then at rest keep the heart rate really low. Much like what the rabbit hunter experienced.

Stay with me here:

We are told our maximum heart rate is 220 minus your age. So if you are 20 years old the fastest your heart should beat is 200. I am 54 so my maximum is 220 − 53 = 167 beats per minute. In August when I turn 55 it will be 165 beats per minute.

Do you get the picture? Every year our hearts are slowing down, which basically means we don't handle stress as well as we did when we were younger.

As we age the heart just cannot beat as fast as it used to. At the same time, the resting heart rate starts creeping up, bringing these two numbers closer together. One of the classic ways of measuring youth, overall health and cardiovascular status is to have a low resting heart rate and a high maximum heart rate.

This is called your "heart rate variability". When you are fit, your heart has the variability to go very high, recover and then beat very low when at rest.

When we were hunting rabbits, we would sprint and get the heart rate up , then rest and be perfectly still while waiting for it to come out of its hole. Once the rabbit was out, the chase was on again and the heart rate goes up, followed by waiting and resting where the heart rate goes very low. This is called Heart Rate Variability Training.

To stay young and healthy we want to have the ability for our heart rate to go up (and catch the rabbit) and then to function at rest with the incredible efficiency of a low resting heart rate. Let's train for exactly that. New research says this can be done in as little as twelve minutes a day![1,2,3] Here's how.

12 Minute Workout
Sprint Recovery Training

This twelve minute routine can be performed daily, or a minimum of three times per week for cardiovascular improvements, or everyday during the Colorado Cleanse. You can use this as your entire workout or as a cardiovascular warm up before yoga, a bike ride or hiking. In these twelve minutes, you will build your cardiovascular base.

Step One: Warm up
Go for a walk, jog, bike ride or use a cardio machine like an elliptical trainer. Exercise slowly for 2 minutes while maximally breathing in and out through

your nose. (In my book *Body, Mind and Sport*, I introduced research on why nasal breathing is important.)

Nasal breathing is a skill that may take some time to master. Don't worry if you have to mouth breath. Do the best you can and – in time – the nasal breathing will get easier.

Step Two: Sprint
Start exercising faster, like a mini sprint for 1 minute. Use the nasal breath during the sprint if you can as it will slow you down and not let you do too much. Don't push it here. Start slow and build yourself up to a faster sprint over time. Try to do a sprint pace that you can maintain for one minute. In a couple of weeks you will be sprinting like a pro.

Step 3: Recovery
Slow the exercise down to the Warm Up pace for one minute and maintain the nasal breathing if you can. Nasal Breathing during the recovery will force air into the lower lobes of the lungs allowing for more efficient release of CO_2 and activation of the calming parasympathetic nervous system that predominates in the lower lobes of the lungs. This will help you release toxins and stress.

Step 4: Second Sprint
Start another sprint for one minute. Make this a little faster if you can. Continue nasal breathing if possible. Sprints can be running up and down stairs, jumping jacks, jumping on and off a curb for one minute – just get the exertion level up.

Step 5: Second Recovery
Recover from the sprint with one minute of deep nasal breathing at the warm up pace. If you cannot maintain nasal breathing during the recovery the sprint was too hard. Each time it will get easier.

Step 6: Continue Sprints and Recoveries
Continue sprints and recoveries for a total of 4 sprints and 4 recoveries. Follow the nasal breathing if you can.

Step 7: Cool Down
Repeat Step 1. Exercise slowing with deep nasal breathing for 2 minutes.

Note: In the beginning you may need a 90 second recovery period after each sprint instead of just one minute. If this is the case then just do a 2 minute warm up, then 3 one minute sprints with 3 90 second recoveries and a 2 minute cool down, for a total of 12 minutes.

Avoid the Dangers of Over Exercising
There is an increasing amount of research indicating the damage of long slow steady training on the heart. In one study 80 marathon runners were tested for the kind of heart damaging chemicals seen after a heart attack. Prior to the marathon runners were free of these chemicals. Right after the marathon and three days later *all* of the runners showed the kind of early stage cardiac damage seen after a heart attack.[4]

It is clear that long, slow duration workouts in your heart rate training zone are not necessary and in some cases can be damaging to your heart. In 12 minutes you can get your cardiovascular base and be free to enjoy a fun bike ride, hike or some yoga. Less has been proven to be more!

Be Calm and Lose Weight
The benefits of this kind of exercise are compelling. Nasal breathing during this workout naturally creates a safe governor for monitoring how much exercise is good and how much more can be potentially harmful, as indicated above.

The sprint/recovery training offers many health benefits (without the wear and tear of a long slow duration workout), such as: [1,2,4]

Increasing fat metabolism.

Calming the nervous system and mind

Stabilizing glucose and insulin levels

Increasing calorie burning

Boosting energy

Creating a sleeker, stronger, and more toned physique

Enhancing sex drive

Improved lymphatic drainage leading to healthier skin and detoxification

Amplifying exercise endurance and performance

Raising growth hormone – which may be responsible for all the above

Heart Rate Variability Training (or Sprint Recovery Training) offers all the benefits of the more strenuous exercise that we have been told to do over the years - but in just 12 minutes!

The Fountain of Youth

When you sprint, fast twitch muscle fibers are activated, which significantly increases muscle circulation and stimulates the production of Human Growth Hormone (HGH). This hormone decreases after 30 years of age and is the fountain of youth if there ever was one. Exercise-induced HGH activation helps restore the youthfulness and elasticity we had in our twenties and alone offers all the benefits of regular exercise.

Take this opportunity to get fit, happy and healthy!

Avoid Injury During Exercise

Too many of my patients tell me that they cannot exercise because they start hurting too bad when they do. They become damned if they exercise and damned if they don't.

Lack of exercise or a sedentary life brews decreased oxygenation of the tissues and poor lymphatic drainage. Basically, the muscles lose blood supply and start to harden. They get stiff and rigid when there is less blood flow because blood is the muscle's lubricant. Without it, the muscles get stiff, strain, inflame and cause pain. When we start exercising with muscles that have lost adequate blood supply they are more likely to strain and tear – leading to injury.

Slowly building up your sprints will help you avoid injuries. Increasing your nasal breathing endurance will also help you handle more exercise because it improves lower lung lobe efficiency. Remember, the lower lobes of the lung are where respiratory waste removal and the calming effects of the parasympathetic nervous system occur.

>>> Learn more:
  ❖ Free Health Report and Video: *"Enjoy Exercise for the First Time Ever!,"* which explains nasal breathing exercise and how to be sure you are not doing too much. www.lifespa.com/breathe.

References:
1. Campbell, Phill, A. Ready Set Go, Pristine Publishers, Inc.
2. Sears, A. PACE: The Twelve Minute Fitness Revolution
3. Roskamm, Canada. Med. Ass. J. Mar. 25,1967, vol. 96 Physical Activity and Cardiovascular Health 895
4. Siegel A., et al. Effect of marathon running on inflammatory and hemostatic markers. *Amer Jour Card*. Volume 88, Number 8, 15 October 2001

Success Story
~ I lost 9 lbs. I feel good and calm. My skin glows, no wrinkles (and I'm 53). I'm in tune with the rhythm of the day. I'm sleeping great. No cravings. I'm a happy camper!!

PART I
GENERAL CLEANSING GUIDELINES
(DAYS 1 – 14)

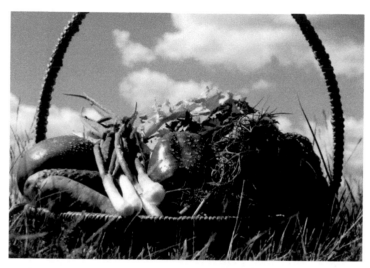

Now that you have an understanding of why it is important to detox and reset the digestion, we can begin! During all phases of the Colorado Cleanse follow these General Guidelines.

The herbal program I suggest will support your body by clearing and strengthening detox channels, optimizing liver and gallbladder function, and helping to heal digestion.

By following the Lifestyle Guidelines you will quiet the mind, unwind the nervous system, and help release old mental and emotional patterns and behaviors.

The dietary guidelines to avoid common allergens will give your digestion a break from hard to digest foods so your body can focus its energy on detox. In addition, this will help your body repair the intestinal mucosa and strengthen digestion.

In the future, after the Colorado Cleanse, you can return to these General Cleansing Guidelines for a few days to reset your system if you are going through a period of feeling run down, stressed, or not eating well.

CHAPTER 6
HERBS TO MAXIMIZE YOUR BENEFITS

I strongly suggest that you take these recommended herbs, which will increase your benefits and make the Colorado Cleanse more comfortable and effective. We sell all of these herbs at LifeSpa separately and in a 'Colorado Cleanse Supply Kit' (see page 161). I always recommend choosing organic or ethically wild crafted whole herbs, rather than concentrates or extracts. I also make suggestions for alternative herbal strategies that are available in your health food store.

As always, listen to your body and adjust your dosage of each herb as needed.

Success Story
~ This cleanse- my second with you- was again a life changing experience. I am now within 5 pounds of my high school graduation weight and I am 56 years old! I had learned that I have celiac disease about 5 months before the last cleanse. I truly felt so awful all the time I wasn't sure how much longer I could go on. I was feeling so sluggish and bloated. The cleanse was just what I needed to undo all those years of poisoning myself! Between changing my diet and repairing my digestive system, I feel like I am living in a different body!

Lymphatic Detox

The lymph system starts on the inside of the intestinal wall as intestinal villi and lacteals, where it pulls fat soluble nutrition and chemicals into the Gut Associated Lymphatic Tissue (GALT), which is the largest concentration of lymph in the body. It is here that we find 80% of the body's immune strength. The integrity of the relationship of the lacteals and villi on the inside of the gut wall and the GALT is one of the most important in the human body. I call this the most important half inch in the human body - and we have miles of it.

The best herbal lymphatic de-stagnator I have found is an herb called *Manjistha* (Rubia cordifolia), pronounced 'man-gee-stuh'. *Manjistha* cleanses the lymph around the gut and all the lymph channels in the body - which is about twice as large as the vast arterial blood supply system. In addition to skin that wraps the outside of your body, you have an inner skin that actually wraps every organ, vessel and cavity on the inside of the body as well. All the skin – both inside and out – drains into the lymphatic system. Making sure the skin is properly drained into a healthy lymphatic system will determine how you look and feel. Eighty percent of what your skin looks like is determined by the function of the lymph and skin on the inside of the body. The lymph that drains the skin is called Skin Associated Lymphatic Tissue (SALT). This is a type of Mucus Membrane Associated Lymphatic Tissue (MALT). Your

Symptoms of Lymphatic Congestion

- Allergies
- Rashes
- Itching skin
- Swollen hands or feet
- Holding onto more water
- PMS
- Breast swelling or tenderness
- Headaches
- Joint pain that moves around the body
- Swelling around the abdomen
- Cellulite
- Breast lumps
- Fibroid tumors
- Ovarian cysts
- Sore feet in the morning
- Sore throats
- Chronic colds
- Weak immunity
- Constipation
- Fatigue
- Lack of mental clarity
- Cold hands and feet

SALT, MALT and GALT are your first line of defense against toxins and infection. In a healthy lymphatic system, you have 25 billion lymphocytes passing through each lymph node each day that help your body process toxins. *Manjistha* plays a crucial role in helping your lymph system function optimally so you can continuously flush out toxins.

The lymphatic system drains the wastes from your body and controls and regulates your immune system. It is pumped through muscular contractions, so if one is sedentary, the lymphatic system will eventually become sedentary as well. This will create toxicity in lymphatic related tissues such as breasts, skin, joints, and muscles. When the lymph system becomes sluggish, you may experience one or more of the Symptoms of Lymphatic Congestion.

Manjistha Dosage

Based on your sensitivity to herbs, take this herb as follows:
- **Please take 500 mg, 3 times per day, after each meal.**
- **Take for 4 weeks starting on Day 1.**
- Most everyone can easily tolerate this herb, but if you are sensitive to herbs then take 500 mg 2 times per day for 6 weeks after meals.
- The only known side effect of *Manjistha* is that, like beets, it may make your urine turn a slight reddish color. This is normal.

LifeSpa's *Manjistha* formula includes Gokshura, which helps drive it deeper into the lymphatic system.

Alternative to Manjistha: Take Red Root tincture, a commonly available herb that helps de-stagnate and detox the lymph and lymph nodes. Take 1 dropperful in warm water after each meal.

>>> Learn More - Free Health Report and Videos:
- *The Miracle of Lymph* at www.lifespa.com/lymph.
- *Feel and Look Vibrant in 3 Steps – The Most Important ½ Inch of Your Body* at www.lifespa.com/skin.

Repair the Villi

There are many factors that are responsible for injuring and irritating the villi such as: stress, overeating, spicy food and coffee in excess, along with exposure to yeast and bacteria. Two things can happen when the mucus membranes of the gut become irritated:

1. They can become dry, which causes constipation.
2. They produce excessive reactive mucus which creates looser stools and compromises the assimilation of nutrients and the detoxification of waste. These villi are really where it all starts. If excess mucus is produced, the villi flatten out and become non-functional.

Turmeric is an herb that helps pull excess reactive mucus off the villi of the intestinal tract and stimulate the flow of lymph which drains the gut. Turmeric also helps thin the bile and decongest the liver.

There are many kinds of digestive imbalances that contribute to a compromised immune system. These include constipation, diarrhea, indigestion, and acid reflux to name a few. Any irritation or inflammation of the gut will affect the function of the villi. The villi are responsible for assimilation of nutrients, immunity and the removal of toxins that are responsible for compromising the immunity.

Here are some of the reports on turmeric's effectiveness:

Turmeric increases immune boosting antioxidant activity by increasing production of glutathione and super oxide dismutase (SOD).[1]

Turmeric, much like vitamin D3, decreases immune compromising inflammatory cytokines that cause lymphatic congestion and a sluggish immune response.[2] Turmeric increases gallbladder function and bile flow. Bile flow in the gut is the intestine's first immune responder against infection. Bile also emulsifies disease producing fat soluble toxins.[3]

Turmeric repairs gastric and duodenal ulcers with the same properties that it helps to heal damaged and inflamed intestinal villi.[4] Non-functional villi compromise immunity.

Turmeric (Curcuma longa) is one of the best herbs to thin the mucus and heal the intestinal skin or epithelium. I recommend a formula that includes black pepper, which - in the proper ratio - has been shown to increase the absorption of turmeric by 2000%.[5] In one study, turmeric with black pepper out-performed chemotherapy drugs for colon cancer. There are numerous studies showing curcumin's ability to match chemotherapy drugs for breast cancer and leukemia.[7]

Turmeric Dosage

Based on your sensitivity to herbs, take this herb as follows:
- ❖ **Please take 500mg, 3 times per day, after each meal.**
- ❖ **Take for 4 weeks, starting on Day 1.**

There are no known side effects for Turmeric.

Most everyone can tolerate this herb, but if you are sensitive to herbs then take 500 mg, 2 times per day for 6 weeks after meals.

LifeSpa carries a formula called *Turmeric Plus*, which includes the proper ratio of black pepper.

Alternative to *Turmeric Plus*: Drink 1 cup of Dandelion Root Tea after each meal. Or, after each meal, mix ¼ teaspoon of turmeric with a dash of black pepper in just enough raw honey to make a paste.

>>> Learn More – Free Health Report and Videos:

❖ *Turmeric Prevents Cancer, Alzheimer's and More* at www.lifespa.com/turmeric.

❖ *Prevent Diabesity – the Next Epidemic* at www.lifespa.com/diabesity, which is about balancing blood sugar.

❖ *The Miracle of Lymph* at www.lifespa.com/lymph.

References

1. J Ethnopharm. 2007 Sep 25;113(3):479-86
2. Life Sci. 2007 Feb. 13;80(10):926-31
3. Rasyid A, Lelo A. The effect of curcumin and placebo on human gall-bladder function: an ultrasound study. *Aliment Pharmacol Ther.* 1999;13:245-249
4. Van Dau N, Ngoc Ham N, Huy Khac D, et al. The effects of a traditional drug, turmeric *(Curcuma longa),* and placebo on the healing of duodenal ulcer. *Phytomedicine.* 1998;5:29-34.
5. St. John's Medical College, 1998, Bangalore, India
6. Mol Cancer Ther. 2007 Apr;6(4):1276-82.
7. Int J Mol Med. 2007 Sep;20(3):329-35

Thin the Bile and Cleanse the Liver

Most of us have intestinal villi that have become congested and lymph that has become sluggish to some degree. This creates a scenario that forces toxins to default back to the liver for detoxification. The problem is that the villi and lymph were designed to take care of the fat soluble toxins that flood our food and environment.   In our modern lives, the liver ends up becoming overwhelmed with its detox responsibilities. The liver will spill these toxins back into the blood and put them in fatty store houses in the body. The two most common areas are the fat cells in the body and in the brain.

I developed a formula called *Liver Repair,* which is designed to repair and cleanse the liver while thinning the bile. When the liver becomes congested, the bile becomes too thick which slows, and sometimes stops, the liver's ability to digest fats as well as it once did. You may have noticed that over the years you tend to avoid foods that are rich or heavy like wheat, gluten, soy, dairy or fried foods. The bile is also designed to emulsify the fat soluble toxins. If the bile is too thick, these toxins never get properly processed. Taking bile thinners is an important part of our cleanse. We need the liver to be decongested and the bile to be thin so the liver can properly process the release of toxins stored in our fatty tissue.

Liver Repair Dosage

Based on your sensitivity to herbs I would like you to take this herb as follows:
  * **Please take 500mg, 3 times per day, after each meal.**
  * **Take for 4 weeks starting on Day 1.**

If you experience any loose stools or digestive discomfort take fewer capsules per day to find the dose that is best for you (even if it is only 1 capsule per day). If we flush the liver too quickly the increased bile flow will loosen the stool. Cleansing does not have to be uncomfortable.

LifeSpa's *Liver Repair* is one of the best herbal formulas to repair and cleanse the liver while thinning the bile. *Liver Repair* is a combination of herbs that cleanse and repair the liver:
  * Bhumy Amalaki – flushes bile through the liver.
  * Picorrhiza – repairs liver damage.
  * Guduchi – liver tonic.
  * Turmeric – thins the bile and protects the liver.
  * Amalaki – repairs damaged tissue and epithelium in the liver and small intestine.

Alternative to *Liver Repair*: Take 250 mg of Milk Thistle three times per day after food.

Flush the Bile Ducts

When the villi of the intestines become irritated and congested, the lymph around the gut also congests. Toxins default back to the liver, making the bile thick and viscous. This thick bile congests the bile and pancreatic ducts, which compromises the ability to digest fats and allow pancreatic enzymes to flow freely into the small intestine. When the bile becomes too viscous and thick, these ducts become congested and the digestion of fats, detoxification of fat soluble toxins and the flow of digestive enzymes become compromised. De-stagnating these ducts is a critical component in increasing fat metabolism, detoxification and stabilizing blood sugar, energy and mood.   Learn   more   at www.lifespa.com/digestivehealth.

Beet Cleanse Dosage

Based on your sensitivity to herbs, take this herb as follows:
- ❖ **Please take 500mg, 3 times per day, 15 minutes before meals with 12 oz of warm water.**
- ❖ **Take for 3 weeks, starting on Day 1.**

Note: During the Post Cleanse, the dose increases on Days 12-19, which is detailed in the Digestive Strength protocol on page 116.

LifeSpa's *Beet Cleanse* is a unique formulation designed to flush stagnant bile from the biliary tubes in the liver and the bile, and the cystic and pancreatic ducts. It contains the following organic ingredients: Beets to increase bile flow and thin the bile; Fenugreek to cleanse the bile and pancreatic ducts and balance blood sugar; Cinnamon to balance blood sugar and increase bile and digestive enzyme flow; and Shilajit to remove congestion in the bile and pancreatic ducts

Alternative to *Beet Cleanse*: Eat more raw beets, 2-3 per day, and drink 1 cup of fenugreek tea after each meal. To make fenugreek tea steep 1 Tbsp of fenugreek seed in hot water for 20 minutes.

Boost Absorption, Mood, Energy and Detox

New research has revealed powerful rejuvenative properties of an herb that Ayurvedic texts labeled a panacea – or cure all – thousands of years ago. This ancient Ayurvedic secret is Shilajit, also known as "the destroyer of weakness."

For thousands of years Shilajit has been used to help:

- ❖ Increase energy.
- ❖ Boost mood.
- ❖ Improve memory.
- ❖ Decrease anxiety.
- ❖ Increase absorption and potency of nutrients.
- ❖ Prevent or treat Alzheimer's, Parkinson's and Diabetes.
- ❖ Balance blood sugar levels.
- ❖ Detoxify heavy metals and toxins from the body.
- ❖ Increase oxygenation and fight free radicals in the cells.
- ❖ Break down cysts and tumors.

For millennia Shilajit has been touted as the best carrier of energy and nutrition into the human body. Modern science has recently proven this by identifying fulvic and humic acids, which are found in abundance in Shilajit, as the main substances responsible for energy production within the cell.[1] Science is just beginning to understand the implications of fulvic acid rich nutrients like Shilajit.

Researchers are excited about Shilajit's unprecedented medicinal potential, such as increasing the potency of other nutrients by up to 30%! In addition to the fulvic acids, Shilajit is like a refrigerator full of many nutrients and minerals. The other primary component of Shilajit is DBP's (dibenzo alpha pyrones) which are the energizer bunny component. This herb delivers more energy than any other, without being a stimulant, and why it is the only herb, out of 2000 medicinal plants, given the label 'panacea' in the Indian Materia Medica.

Shilajit is the Essence of Ancient Tropical Forests

About 40 million years ago, the Indian continent collided into Asia and formed the Himalayan mountain range. Tropical forests were crushed and compacted between massive boulders as the mountains formed. The compressed forests gradually transformed into a nutrient and mineral rich biomass loaded with medicinal humic and fulvic acids. Every summer as the mountains warm, India's most powerful medicine literally exudes from these biomass resins in high mountain crevices.

Renew Your Cells

It is well known that highly oxygenated cells are resistant to cancer, cell death and disease. Shilajit is heralded as a panacea because of its ability to actually regenerate a cell by driving oxygen and nutrients into the cell[5] and push damaging free radicals out of the cell.[6] It is for this reason that I named our new Shilajit product "*Regenerate*."

Have you ever wondered how a plant pulls minerals out of the soil and transforms them into a bio-available nutrient for the plant? Or how minerals are delivered into a cell in the body? Fulvic acid is what makes both these processes possible. Shilajit is one of the richest sources of fulvic acid in the world.

Shilajit Makes all Herbs and Nutrients More Effective

Have you heard of "colloidal minerals"? They are minerals in solution that are much easier to absorb than other mineral supplements. Yes - it is the fulvic acids found in Shilajit that bring minerals we so desperately need into a colloidal solution. Once in solution we can digest and assimilate the minerals.

Traditionally, Shilajit was described as "yoga vahi" which means that whatever it is taken with will be enhanced due to Shilajit's ability to bring any nutrient into solution and drive it into the cell.

In one study CoQ10, which boosts energy in heart, liver and kidney cells, was enhanced by 29% with the addition of Shilajit.[2]

Feeling Tired? No Endurance?

Shilajit is one of the most amazing herbs for deep rejuvenation and energy production. In a recent study participants took just 200mg of Shilajit each day for 15 days and the available energy in their blood after vigorous exercise was equivalent to the levels of available energy before starting exercise.[4]

Recent studies on Shilajit show that it delivers energy and nutrients to the cell at astonishing levels. In one study mice underwent strenuous exercise and had their energy (ATP) expenditure measured with and without Shilajit. The energy depleted twice as fast with the group that did not take the Shilajit.[3]

Mood Support: Shilajit increases dopamine in the brain. Dopamine is a neurotransmitter that is responsible for feelings of contentment and is a possible treatment for Parkinson's disease.[7]

Memory: Shilajit improves learning acquisition and memory retrieval by driving oxygen, minerals and nutrients into the brain tissue while protecting the brain from neuro toxins.[8]

Anxiety: Shilajit reduces anxiety.[8] Anxiety is caused by a state of exhaustion where there is not enough energy to sedate and calm the nervous system. Shilajit rebuilds the energy reserves.

Super Anti-Oxidant: Shilajit dramatically increases levels of powerful anti-oxidants, such as Glutathione peroxidase and Super oxide dismutase and Catalase, in brain tissue. which protects the brain from oxidative damage and cognitive decline.[9]

Blood Sugar: Shilajit lowers fasting blood sugar, providing stable energy, improved mood, better fat metabolism and decreased cravings.[12]

Inflammation: Shilajit reduces inflammation by driving oxygen to the cells and increasing antioxidant activity. [12]

Diabetes: Shilajit protects pancreatic cells from diabetes by increasing antioxidant activity and regenerating cellular energy and repair.[10]

Alzheimer's Disease: Shilajit protects neurotransmitters in the brain that may help prevent Alzheimer's disease. [11]

Detoxification: Fulvic acids found in Shilajit are very porous, allowing nutrition and energy to be carried into the cell and toxins to be pulled out of the cells. [13, 14]

As the most powerful natural electrolyte known, fulvic acid restores electrical balance to damaged cells, neutralizes toxins and can eliminate food poisoning within minutes. [13, 14]

Cysts and Tumors: Traditionally, Shilajit has been used to break up cysts and tumors, such as ovarian, liver and breast cysts, and malignant or benign tumors.

Shilajit Dosage

Based on your sensitivity to herbs I would like you to take this herb as follows:
- ❖ **Take 300 mg of Shilajit, 3 times per day after meals.**
- ❖ **Take for 4 weeks starting on Day 1.**

LifeSpa's Shilajit *Regenerate* formula follows the recommendation of Ayurvedic doctors to further maximize Shilajit's effectiveness by combining it with small amounts of Ashwaganda and Amalaki - two incredible herbs in their own right.

Alternatives to Shilajit: Shilajit is a rare herb and hard to replace. Adaptogens like ginseng, astragalas or rhodiola will provide excellent rejuvenation.

References:
1. Agarwal SP, Khanna R, Karmarkar R, Anwer MK, Khar RK. Shilajit: a review. Phytother Res. 2007 May;21(5):401-5.
2. Bhattacharyya S, Pal D, Banerjee D, et al. Shilajit dibenzo—pyrones: Mitochondria targeted antioxidants. Pharmacologyonline. 2009; 2:690-8.
3. Bhattacharyya S, Pal D, Gupta AK, Ganguly P, Majumder UK, Ghosal S. Beneficial effect of processed shilajit on swimming exercise induced impaired energy status of mice. Pharmacologyonline. 2009;1:817-25.

4. Pal D, Bhattacharya S. Pilot Study on the Improvement of Human Performance with ReVitalETTM as Energy Booster: Part-IV. 2006. Data on file. Natreon, Inc.

5. Visser SA. Effect of humic substances on mitochondrial respiration and oxidative phosphorylation. Sci Total Environ. 1987 Apr;62:347-54.

6. Piotrowska D, Dlugosz A, Witkiewicz K, Pajak J. The research on antioxidative properties of TOLPA Peat Preparation and its fractions. Acta Pol Pharm. 2000 Nov;57 Suppl:127-9.

7,8,9,10,11. Ghosal S. Shilajit in Perspective. Oxford, U.K.: Narosa Publishing House; 2006

12. Clinical study for evaluation of plasma antioxidant capacity and safe use of purified and standardized Shilajit (ReVitalET) in normal volunteers. J. B. Roy State Ayurvedic Medical College and Hospital, Kolkata. 2007. Data on file. Natreon, Inc.

13. Paraquat - Fischer, A.M., Winterie, J.S., Mill, T. (1967). Primary photochemical processes in photolysis medicated by humic substances. In R.G. Zika, W.J. Cooper (Eds). Photochemistry of environmental aquatic system (141-156). (ACS Symposium Series 327). Washington D.C.: American Chemical Society.

14. Pesticides - Aiken, G.R. McKnight, D.M. MacCarthy, P. (1985). Humic substances of soil, sediment and water. New York: Wiley-Interscience

Balance Blood Sugar

If eating 3 meals a day presents a challenge or you just can't seem to muster the will power to give up the dark chocolate, coffee or jelly beans because your cravings are just out of control, let me introduce you to an herb that is nothing short of amazing.

Gymnema sylvestre is an Ayurvedic herb from the milkweed family that is locally known as Gurmar or the *"Sugar Destroyer."* If you put just a taste of this herb on your tongue and then ate a candy bar or anything with sugar, you simply would not taste the sugar. It literally blocks the absorption of the sugar through the taste buds and the intestinal wall.[1] The active ingredients, gymnemic acids, have receptors both in the gut and on the tongue aiding in blocking sugar absorption. When sugar absorption is blocked, cravings are reduced and blood sugar highs and lows are neutralized. If sugar is blocked at both points of entry the body must get its energy elsewhere. Fat is mobilized as the fuel supply of choice. *Sugar Destroyer* resets the body's ability to use fat as fuel rather than sugar or carbohydrates.

LifeSpa's *Sugar Destroyer* formula also helps to stabilize blood sugar levels and makes the transition from six meals a day to three doable - and even preferable.

In one study, Gymnema was administered for 18 to 20 months to 22 Type II diabetics taking conventional medication. All patients showed a significant reduction in blood glucose levels. Five of the 22 maintained their blood glucose levels without conventional drugs and the dose of the medications were reduced in the others.[2,3]

Sugar Destroyer is a harmonizer for the blood sugar and pancreas. It balances both high blood sugar, as in diabetes, and low blood sugar, as in hypoglycemia. In natural medicine this is called "herbal intelligence" because it has the ability to bring balanced function to the pancreas and blood sugar rather than just reduce symptoms.

Gymnema Dosage

Based on your sensitivity to herbs, take this herb as follows:
- ❖ **Take 500mg, 3 times per day 15 minutes before meals, with 12oz of warm water.**
- ❖ **Take for 4 weeks starting on Day 1.**

Even if you think you do not have a blood sugar imbalance I highly recommend that you follow this protocol to ensure a strong and healthy pancreas.

LifeSpa's *Sugar Destroyer* is Gymnema, combined with *Shilajit*, which is rich in fulvic acids and helps reduce insulin resistance based cravings by helping carry insulin and sugar into resistant cells, thus stabilizing blood sugar.

Alternative to *Sugar Destroyer*: Drink cinnamon tea. Steep a cinnamon stick in hot water for 20 minutes and drink 1 cup 15 minutes before meals.

References:
1. Shimizu K et al. *J VetMed* Sci 1997; 59:245
2. Baskaran K et al. Antidiabetic effect of a leaf extract from Gymnema sylvestre in   noninsulin-dependent diabetes mellitus patients. *J Ethnopharmacoll990;* 30:295
3. Shanmugasundaram ER. et al. Use of Gynrnema sylvestre leaf extract in the control of blood glucose in insulin-dependent diabetes mellitus. *J Ethnopharmacoll990;* 30:281

Increase Digestive Strength

Digestive Enzymes are OK - for the Short Term and in Small Doses

The issue with enzymes is not that they are "bad" -- they have a place in supporting a digestive imbalance for *short periods of time*. Like any medicine - you get on it, get better, and then get off. Even if you are taking small dosages of enzymes, this is a sign that your digestion is weak and will only continue to get weaker unless you strengthen it.

Unfortunately, we are told that our bodies do not make these enzymes after a certain age and that they are needed long term to make up for this lack. I do not believe this. The digestive system can be reset to produce adequate amounts of enzymes and not need any supplementation for maintaining good digestion. It is the misunderstanding that we need digestive enzymes forever that I am concerned about because they create long term dependency and weaken your digestion. For the short term digestive enzymes can be useful - as long as you have an exit strategy.

At LifeSpa I use two herbs in my clinical practice to reset and increase digestive strength. *Warm Digest* is for boggy digestion and *Cool Digest* for hyperacidity.

Warm Digest Knowledge

Warm Digest is taken before meals to stimulate the digestive enzymes that the body naturally produces. What I have found practicing natural medicine and Ayurveda for 22 years is that Digestive Enzymes are handed out like Gatorade for just about any and all digestive imbalances. What folks don't realize is that once you get on them – it is very difficult to get off them.

A few years ago I was honored to lecture with one of the most brilliant natural medicine doctors of our time. He was in his nineties and after writing 50 books, developing iridology and colon cleansing therapy, I was told he was taking 17 digestive enzymes with every meal. This was due to excessive intestinal cleansing and colonics. To the "rescue" came digestive enzymes which do the digesting for you. They helped him digest his food and slowly but surely he needed more and more of them until he was forced to take 17 with each meal.

While there is a time and place for enzymes as a medicine for short term use to help your digestion in an emergency, long term use is not in your best interest. Regular use of digestive enzymes weakens digestion because your body no longer has to do the work itself and you will then become dependent on them. Similar to exercise, if you stop exercising you start to atrophy and become weak.

Ayurvedic medicine is designed to restore body balance so the body can heal itself without dependence on pills or powders. My goal with all my patients is to get them well, often with the use of herbs. As soon as we reach a clinically effective dose, I start to wean them off that herb so we don't create such dependencies. In Ayurveda there is a classic remedy for the digestive process called trikatu. Trikatu actually resets the ability for you to digest your own food rather than do the digesting for you. LifeSpa's *Warm Digest* is comprised of trikatu, which is a simple combination of Ginger, Black Pepper and Long Pepper:

- ❖ Ginger is perhaps one of the world's finest digestive aids that won't overheat the digestive process.
- ❖ Black pepper stimulates the flow of your own digestive enzymes.
- ❖ Long pepper helps to strengthen the digestion and break down hard to digest foods - and like ginger it won't overheat the digestive process.

I love *Warm Digest* because it can help restore normal and healthy digestive function so you can steadily wean off it - when combined with an understanding of How, When and What to eat - like I talk about in my book *The 3-Season Diet*.

Cool Digest Knowledge

Combining fennel, guduchi, cumin and other spices, *Cool Digest* is extremely effective for kindling digestive ability while cooling the irritated mucosa of the stomach wall. It counteracts excessive stomach acid production. *Cool Digest* cools and strengthens the digestive system. Under stress, the digestive system produces excessive amounts of acids, which overheat the system and strip the mucus lining from the stomach wall, weakening digestion, heating and ulcerating the wall of stomach and/or upper intestinal lining. For any weak digestive system or a system that is experiencing ulceration, heat, heartburn or indigestion, *Cool Digest* is a better choice.

Warm Digest or Cool Digest Dosage

If you ever experience acid reflux or heartburn after eating meals that are heavy, rich, or late in the evening, take *Cool Digest*. Otherwise take *Warm Digest*, which is appropriate for the majority of people.

Based on your sensitivity to herbs, take this herb as follows:
- ❖ **Take 500 mg of *Warm Digest* or *Cool Digest*, 3 times per, day 15 minutes before meals, with 12oz of warm water.**
- ❖ **Take for 3 weeks starting on Day 1.**
- ❖ Notes: On Day 12, during the Post Cleanse, the dosage increases. Follow the Digestive Strength Protocol on page 116.

Alternatives to *Warm Digest*: Take 500 mg of Trikatu before meals or chew 2 slices of 'ginger pizza' 15 minutes before meals. To make 'ginger pizza': slice fresh, raw, peeled ginger root into thin rounds. Sprinkle with lemon juice and sea salt. You can make enough to last a few days and simply store them in the fridge.

Alternative to *Cool Digest*: Drink one cup of hot water mixed with a pinch of ginger, cumin and fennel powder. Drink with your meals.

CHAPTER 7
LIFESTYLE GUIDELINES FOR DAYS 1 - 14

Follow the Below Guidelines for the Entire Two Week Cleanse.

Do the best you can! The following guidelines will greatly enhance the effectiveness of the Colorado Cleanse, but are not required.

Daily Tools for Unwinding the Nervous System

I co-produced 3 DVDs with Gaiam which all include a daily practice for Yoga, Breathing, Self-Massage, Exercise with Nasal Breathing and Meditation. Each DVD focuses on a specific goal: *Ayurveda for Stress, Ayurveda for Detox* or *Ayurveda for Weight Loss.*

 The DVDs are a great resource during – and after – the Colorado Cleanse. If you do not have one of these DVDs I have listed alternatives below.

To improve lymphatic flow and calm the mind, practice the following 5 stress relief techniques every day.

Yoga
(10-15 minutes per day)

Follow one of these gentle yoga routines for 10-15 minutes every day:
* ❖ *Ayurveda for Stress* DVD: Restorative
* ❖ *Ayurveda for Detox* DVD: Lymph Flow
* ❖ *Ayurveda for Weight Loss* DVD: Fat Burning
* ❖ Sun Salutations on page 139.

Q: I currently practice yoga at home. Should I stick with my current practice/poses, or should I rather try to do Dr. John's yoga poses in the DVD?

A: The poses in the *Ayurveda for Detox DVD* are Ayurvedically designed to support detox and stimulate the flow of prana and lymph. The long holds will activate the subtle energy system that is designed to enhance normal physiological function and release old molecules of emotion that can hold us hostage to old mental and emotional patterns.

Q: I woke up this morning feeling pretty achy, particularly in my hips and thighs. When I did the yoga practice I really felt discomfort in my thighs and particularly in my hamstrings, can you suggest why this is happening?
A: You may just be sore from the yoga and may take a couple of days to gear up. This could also be due to a cleansing effect. As we start the Main Cleanse you should begin to feel lighter.

Breathing
(5-10 minutes, 1-2 times per day).

Breathing, also known as Pranayama, can be a balancing way to start and end each day. Follow the breathing technique on your Gaiam DVD for 5-10 minutes at least once per day, and ideally twice per day. You can do the Breathing practices anytime of the day that works best for you.

If you do not have the Gaiam DVD, you can do Alternate Nostril Breathing:
1. Inhale through your right nostril, with left nostril closed.
2. Exhale through your left nostril, with right nostril closed.
3. Inhale through your left nostril, with your right nostril closed.
4. Exhale through your right nostril, with left nostril closed.

❖ Inhale and exhale with deep, long, slow breaths.
❖ Continue this pattern for 5-10 minutes.
❖ To close your nostril, hold it gently closed with your finger: with your right hand, use your thumb to close your right nostril and your middle finger to close your left nostril. This makes it easy to smoothly alternate nostrils.

Abhyanga Self-Massage
(1-20 minutes per day)

Daily self-massage is a powerful technique to calm and disarm the nervous system while activating detoxification pathways. You can do your self-massage for just 1-3 minutes during or after a shower. Though Ayurveda traditionally recommends that you do self-massage in the morning, you can do it whenever it is most convenient for you. For instructions on how to do daily self- massage, please refer to your *Ayurveda for Detox* DVD or page 141.

Exercise with Nasal Breathing
(12 minutes per day)

At least 12 minutes each day, choose exercises you enjoy such as walking, jogging, hiking, cycling, or dancing. Try these with my interval technique in *Be Fit in 12 minutes a Day* on page 37.

If you are not familiar with how to incorporate nasal breathing into your exercise routine, please refer to the exercise section on your Gaiam DVD, or refer to my Health Report archives at www.lifespa.com/news.

>>> Learn More:
   ❖ Read my book *Body, Mind and Sport.*

Meditation
(10-20 minutes, 1-2 times per day)

Meditate 1-2 times per day for 10-20 minutes. Many people like to meditate first thing in the morning and again before bed.

Follow the Meditation Practice on your Gaiam DVD. If you already have a meditation practice that works well for you, please continue.

How to do My One Minute Meditation:

If you do not have one of the DVDs and do not already have a meditation practice, follow my *One Minute Meditation*. It pumps oxygen into your brain so your brain begins to feel from the heart rather than think from the mind. You can watch a YouTube video of the One Minute Meditation at www.lifespa.com/meditatation.

This is a wonderful meditation for relief of anxiety. It starts with pumping oxygen into your brain, with deep nasal bellows breathing, followed by sitting quietly with your eyes closed. You start with about 30 seconds of Bellows Breathing, and follow that with about 30 seconds of silence with eyes closed. This pumps enough energy into your nervous system to give you the ability to be more calm and settle your mind.

Bellows Breath
Breathe deep through your nose, in and out, using all five lobes of your lungs like they are a big bellows. You can do this with your eyes closed. Expand and relax your lungs in and out as much as you can while breathing in and out only through your nose, not through your mouth.

Our upper lungs have stress receptors that get activated when our breath is shallow, which is how most of us breathe throughout the day. When we use our lower lungs, like in Bellows Breath, we activate calm receptors that soothe our nervous system.

Extended Meditation
If you would like to meditate longer, you can start by doing Bellows Breath for 30 seconds.

Then sit quietly with your eyes closed until you start thinking again. When you feel thoughts resurfacing, do Bellows Breath again for 10-20 seconds to quiet your mind.

Sit quietly again until thoughts arise and follow once again with Bellows Breath for 10-20 seconds.

Follow this cycle until you feel you are done meditating.

Eat 3 Meals a Day – No Snacking

If you find it difficult to eat 3 meals a day without snacking due to blood sugar levels, please read this section.

In the past ten years we have been told that eating many small meals throughout the day is better than three. Let me explain why this advice is flawed. When you eat 6 meals a day the body takes all of its energy from each meal with no need to draw energy from your reserves, which is your fat. Why would the body burn fat when it is fed every 2-3 hours with a snack – even if it's healthy?

If you want to burn fat - and you do, because burning fat does way more than just make you lose weight - you have to give the body a reason to burn the fat. If you eat breakfast and nothing else until lunch, you will burn fat in between those meals. If you have a carrot as a snack in between these meals you will burn the carrot. It is not bad, you just didn't burn any fat that day.

Why You Want to Become a Fantastic Fat Burner:
 ❖ It helps you naturally maintain a healthy weight.
 ❖ It is a calm fuel – when it burns you feel relaxed.
 ❖ It is non-emergency, stress-reducing fuel that tells your body the war is over.
 ❖ It neutralizes disease producing acids that are created from excess stress.
 ❖ It detoxifies fat soluble cancer causing chemicals that can store for 20+ years in fat cells.
 ❖ It detoxifies fat soluble molecules of emotion that lock us into repetitive patterns of emotional behaviors that cause stress and disease.
 ❖ It stimulates lymphatic drainage.

How to Transition to 3 Meals a Day
 ❖ If you are used to grazing or eating more than 3 meals a day, start with eating 4 meals and work towards 3 meals a day.
 ❖ Make each meal count by stopping to relax and enjoy each meal.
 ❖ Eat enough at breakfast to carry you through to lunch.

❖ Eat a big, warm, satisfying lunch between 10am – 2pm.
Eat enough at lunch to carry you through to supper.

❖ Eat an early and light supper. Eat enough at supper to carry you through the night until breakfast. Think of supper as "supplemental."

Sometimes, we are not really aware of how we self medicate throughout the day until we challenge the blood sugar to go without those sweets. Breaking these patterns is a part of the Colorado Cleanse and a necessary task.

If you are having extreme difficulty with this and you are not able to stop grazing and find it impossible to go without your snack or sweet of choice, the herbal formula, *Sugar Destroyer*, *Regenerate,* and *Beet Cleanse*, which are part of this cleanse, will help you make this transition more gracefully. These herbs have been studied to reset the islet cells of the pancreas to produce insulin and stabilize blood sugar. This is sometimes necessary to help the body balance the blood sugar and make way for an effective cleanse.

During the Colorado Cleanse it can be a little tricky to know how much to eat at each meal because the foods we are eating are more austere than usual. It is common to eat too much in the beginning until you get the flow of eating less.

"If you eat standing up, death looks over your shoulder."
~ *Old Vedic Saying*

One of the most important components of digestion is how we eat. Make the extra effort to sit down, relax and enjoy each meal. Refrain from reading, talking on the phone, checking your email or watching TV. Though it may feel strange at first, your food will begin to taste better, you will eat less and be calmer.

Q: My normal schedule is that I eat breakfast (around 8am), lunch (around noon), then workout after work before going home and eating dinner around 7-8pm. I will need a snack to get me through my workout. Would you recommend a snack? I've made my lunches bigger but I don't like to feel overly full through the afternoon.

A: Yes the big lunches will help, as will more water in the afternoon. Most workouts don't require a snack unless it is very long. A bigger lunch, if the digestive fire is optimal, will last you with more energy into the workout. Remember, as your blood sugar balances and you become an even better fat burner, your need for a snack will slowly disappear.

>>> Learn More:
- ❖ Free Health Report and Video: *3 Meals a Day* at www.lifespa.com/meals.
- ❖ Free Health Report and Video: *How to Prevent Cravings Permanently* at www.lifespa.com/cravings.
- ❖ Read my book *The 3-Season Diet.* www.lifespa.com/3seasondiet.

Rehydration Therapy

Probably the most common cause of digestive problems, lymph congestion and poor detoxification function is due to dehydration. The body, when young and healthy, is up to 80% water. As we age and degenerate we can get as low as 50% water. Hydration is crucial for maintaining optimal health. Once dehydration sets in, it is difficult to rehydrate without special care.

I have had great success combining these two hydration therapies:

Sip Plain Hot Water (Boiled) Every 10-15 Minutes
Boil the water you want to drink for the day for 10 minutes. You can carry a thermos with you to make it easy.

This is an ancient Ayurvedic method for flushing the lymphatic system, softening hardened tissues, and dilating, cleansing and then hydrating deep tissues. It also heals and repairs the digestive system and flushes the GALT (lymph on the outside of the intestinal wall).

Why Boil?: When you boil water, you boil off the dissolved mineral solids in the water, making it much more easy to absorb into the cell. Our cells have aquaporins, which are pores to absorb only H_2O. Distilling or boiling water is the best way to get pure water and nothing else. Boiling also makes the molecules very active, which is why hot water cleanses things better than cold water. The hot water also creates vaso-dilation where the pores and tissues open and thus stimulates better circulation and hydration. The lymph system is rejuvenated by this heating and stimulating effect as well.

Sound Impossible?: Commit to sipping hot water for just one day. But do it well. If you crave more hot water at the end of the day, you are dehydrated. Knowing this, you will likely be more motivated to do it for a full two weeks.

In Addition, Each Day Drink ½ Your Ideal Body Weight in Ounces
For example, if you weigh 120 pounds, drink 60 ounces per day. If you weight 160 lbs but your ideal body weight is 120 pounds, drink 60 ounces per day

Sip plain room temperature water.

This is *in addition* to sipping plain hot water every 10-15 minutes. Do the best you can to drink as much water as possible during the cleanse to moves lymph, increase detox and strengthen digestion.

Q: Does it have to be hot water? I'm hot all the time (pitta, peri-menopause).
A: Please give the hot water a try. As it rehydrates you nd stimulates lymph flow, your body will dissipate the heat much better. This, along with drinking glasses of room temp water, will be the best rehydration technique, and the best way to help your body remove the heat.

Q: Can I have herbal teas between meals?
A: It is best to have herbal teas *with* meals. It is ideal to sip plain warm-to-hot water as much as possible because it is more hydrating and detoxifying for the lymphatic system.

Q: Can I drink ice water?

A: Preferably not. Ice water constricts the vessels of the circulatory system and compromises hydration and the lymphatic system.

Q: I understand the concept of sipping more warm to hot water on the cleanse, but doesn't too much water cool or even extinguish digestive fire and thin digestive juices?
A: Yes, this large amount of water will dilute digestive juices if taken with the meal. You can sip some hot water with the meal and drink a large glass of water 15-20 minutes before the meal - but not during the meal.

Be Gluten-, Dairy-, Allergen- and Sugar- Free

Avoid Gluten (Basically Wheat, Bread and Pasta)

When the stomach acids are not up to par, hard-to-digest gluten can be left undigested in the stomach. During this cleanse, avoid the foods listed in the table at the right. In the last stage of the Colorado Cleanse we will restart the digestive fire and make it easier for you to process hard-to-digest foods like gluten.

❖   **Grain alternatives include:**
    amaranth, quinoa, millet, rice, potatoes, or rice cakes.
❖   Please avoid gluten-free bread and crackers during the cleanse because they are still processed and heavy to digest.

>>> Learn More:
    ❖ Read Chapter 4 *Secrets to Enjoying Gluten Again.*

Avoid Gluten

- Barley
- Bulgur
- Couscous
- Durum
- Einkorn
- Kamut
- Malt
- Oats are usually OK but look for a brand that says, "not contaminated with wheat" or "Certified Gluten-Free"
- Semolina
- Spelt
- Triticale
- Rye
- Wheat
- Wheat bran
- Wheat germ
- Wheat starch

Avoid Dairy

The protein casein in dairy products is hard-to-digest and acts much like gluten does if it is not broken down in the stomach. While we heal and repair the intestinal villi and restart the digestive fire we have to avoid the harder-to-digest foods.

Q: Is it okay to eat dairy on this cleanse? The General Cleansing Guidelines say to avoid dairy, but the Grocery Lists includes some spring dairy products.

A: We included nonfat dairy on the Grocery List in case any of you are in a situation - such as a restaurant or at a friend's - where food choices are limited but you need to stabilize your blood sugar. Nonfat dairy is an acceptable source of protein. If you do eat dairy, we recommend keeping it to small amounts of nonfat yoghurt or nonfat goat's milk. However, please do your best to refrain from eating dairy at all.

>>> Learn More: Read *Don't Eat Dairy Until You Read This!* In Chapter 3.

Avoid Dairy

- Butter
- Yoghurt
- Cottage Cheese
- Cheese
- Milk
- Lactose

Avoid Common Allergens

Hard-to-digest proteins are the cause of 90% of all allergies. During the cleanse it is important that they are avoided because they are potential irritants to the intestinal villi. The eight foods listed in the *Avoid Common Allergens* sidebar at right are required by law to be identified on labels by The Food Allergen Labeling and Consumer Protection Act.

- ❖ Lean meats can be eaten during the cleanse if your blood sugar is unstable.
- ❖ Miso (a soybean product) is okay.

Avoid Common Allergens

- Gluten and Dairy (already mentioned)
- Eggs
- Fish
- Shellfish
- Nuts (seeds are ok)
- Peanuts
- Soy, soybeans

Q: You did not mention any red meats, beef broth, etc. Should I stay away from it totally and be vegetarian/vegan during the cleanse?
A: Yes, this is best. That being said, if a little lean meat will help stabilize your blood sugar and make the cleanse more comfortable, then this is a very acceptable meal.

Q: How about flax seed oil / Fish-oil supplements during the Pre-and Post-Cleanse?
A: It is preferable to avoid these. Get your oils naturally from the seeds, avocadoes, fruits and veggies.

Q: How come no fish? Many are low fat and it is an easy to digest protein.
A: The reality is that fish are unreliable in terms of toxic exposure, such as heavy metals. I wouldn't pick any bones about eating some low fat fish if needed to stabilize blood sugar, if a person were adverse to chicken or red meat.

Protocol: Avoid Sweeteners

Avoid all sweeteners except raw honey in small amounts. Raw honey helps the body mobilize and burn fat so it is an acceptable sweetener while cleansing. (Stevia in small amounts is okay too).

Avoid Sweeteners

- Sugar
- Fructose
- Corn Syrup
- Maple Syrup
- Pasteurized Honey
- Glucose
- Artificial Sweeteners
- Low or no cal sweeteners

If you are having a very strong desire for something sweet, try these tricks:
- ❖ Drink herbal tea with raw honey.
- ❖ Drink ginger tea with lemon and raw honey.
- ❖ Drink broth made of miso or low-sodium veggie broth.
- ❖ To prevent future cravings, be fully relaxed and calm while you eat. Do not watch TV, read, or talk on the phone. This will help your body remember that it has eaten a good, fulfilling meal.
- ❖ Increase your dosage of *Sugar Destroyer* to 2 capsules before meals.
- ❖ Read *Balance Blood Sugar* on page 58 and *Low Blood Sugar?* on page 77.

Caffeine and Nicotine Detox

This is a great time to stop an addiction to caffeine. While this is never an easy task, it will be easier while your body is being compelled to burn fat. Here are a couple of tricks for getting off coffee, cigarettes or other caffeine addictions:

1. Suck on cardamom pods throughout the day. This offers the same taste sensation and antidotes the effect of caffeine.
2. Be sure to follow the Hydration Therapy guidelines in this cleanse.
3. Make each meal really count and don't leave the table unsatisfied.
4. If you get a headache, put a cold ice pack on your head and hot water bottles on your feet for twenty minutes. This vaso-dilates the vessels in the feet and constricts the inflamed vessels in the head. This can be miraculous way to get rid of a headache

Q: Is Black Tea or Green Tea okay?
A: Even black and green tea can be addictive. They are much better than coffee and not irritating to the bowel. If you feel like you can't get through your day without caffeinated tea, that may mean you are exhausted and using the tea to stimulate your body to make energy you don't have. Focus on weaning off by drinking one cup of water before and after your tea and gradually using tea with less and less caffeine. If you are going to have caffeinated tea, have it with food, preferably at lunch, rather than on an empty stomach.

Q: Can I drink coffee on the cleanse? Is it really that bad for me?
A: If you are addicted to coffee this a great time to break the habit if you are up for it. With the cleanse, the bile will be flowing and this will be the easiest time to do it. If you cannot, then do your best to cut back. Drink 8 ounces of water before and after each cup. Try to have it with meals and not on an empty stomach. Brewing it with cardamom also helps protect the gut and neutralize the caffeine. Green tea is a good replacement as needed. Good luck!

Q: Is it okay to have a cup of organic decaf coffee during the cleanse?
A: No, decaf coffee is more dehydrating than regular coffee. The key to the Main Cleanse is to heal the gut and this would defeat the purpose.

CHAPTER 8
SOLUTIONS TO COMMON QUESTIONS

Constipated?

Top 5 Strategies for Relieving Constipation:
1. Take LifeSpa's *Elim I* herbal formula (more details directly below).
   * ❖ An alternative to *Elim I* is trifala (also called triphala), which you can find at most health food stores.
2. Make sure you are following the Rehydration Therapy on page 69.
3. Do at least a little yoga everyday to tone and massage the abdominal region.
4. Eat an early and light dinner.
5. Are you eating enough fiber in the form of vegetables? During the Pre- and Post- Cleanse eat the Beet Salad and Green Smoothie every day, in addition to any vegetables on the current seasonal grocery list.

Q: I am feeling very constipated. I didn't order the Elim I initially. As it will take a few days to receive Elim I in the mail, what should I do?
A: Add some prunes to the khichadi and cook them into it. This is an indication that the villi of the gut are not in the greatest shape and our goal is to get them healthy again. Some of that will take place in the Post Cleanse as well.

Q: Can we do enemas during the cleanse?
A: I'm not a big fan of every day enemas. But if you think you need it on a given day, go ahead and do that. You can also take *Elim I* to help keep the bowels moving. Make sure you are sipping your warm to hot water every 15 minutes.

Q: Help, I'm still having problems with constipation. I took the castor oil on the last night, started taking Trifala, and drinking more water and still nothing.
A: For anyone having problems with constipation, start by increasing your water intake. You can add some chia seeds after meals. Take 1 Tbsp of chia seeds in 8 ounces of water, stir and let sit for 1-2 minutes then drink. Add prunes to your diet as well. If this doesn't help, start taking *Trifala* or *Elim 1*: 2-6 capsules

first thing in the morning and right before bed. If you're still not seeing results you can increase the dosage of *Liver Repair* and *Beet Cleanse* from 3 a day to 4. If still nothing, increase the *Liver Repair* to 5 the next day. As the bowels start moving you can wean off the herbs. Exercise is also important in regulating bowel movements, so try to fit in a walk, jog, bike ride, or some yoga.

Q: I'm taking the Elim I but am not sure I am doing it correctly. What is the protocol?
A: Start by taking 2 capsules first thing in the morning and 2 capsules before bed at night.

1. If you do not move your bowels early the next day, take 3 capsules in the am and pm.
2. Continue increasing daily until you start eliminating once a day in the morning. The maximum dose is 6 capsules in the am and 6 in the pm.
3. Once you start eliminating 1-2 times per day, stay at that dose in the am and pm for a two week period.
4. Slowly Wean Off: After two weeks, if elimination is still once in the morning, gradually reduce the dosage by 1 capsule in the am and pm for two more weeks.
   a. Continue decreasing your dosage by 1 capsule in the am and pm every two weeks.
   b. If you become constipated again, increase to the previous dose for 2 weeks. Once your are elimination once in the morning again, then start decreasing your dosage.

Q: Can I take a natural laxative to relieve constipation, like senna or cascara sagrada?
A: These herbal laxatives are bowel irritants which irritate, dehydrate and desensitize the intestinal mucosa. They will get you to go but are habit forming and problematic. Our goal is to heal the villi and these are very harsh on the gut wall. Use them as a last resort. Magnesium is better but still dehydrates the bowel.

>>> Learn More: See my Free Health Report and Video on natural laxatives at www.lifespa.com/constipation.

Headaches?

Q: Do you expect that some people may get headaches on this cleanse? If you see people get "cleansing reactions", do you have some advice for relief? I want to avoid migraines.

A: Actually, because we are preparing the detox channels and balancing blood sugar before we start the main cleanse - headaches are uncommon unless one is not hydrated, which we have covered, or if they are detoxing from something like coffee, chocolate or cigarettes. In this case you can place a cool ice cloth on the forehead and put heat on the feet for 20-30 minutes. This is an amazing technique to remove detox withdrawal symptoms.

Low Blood Sugar?

If you are feeling unusually moody, groggy, weak, or fatigued, you may be experiencing symptoms of low blood sugar. While cleansing, if the blood sugar is crashing, the body will go into chemical survival and start storing fat. This will defeat the purpose of the cleanse, which is to release toxins stored in fat cells and switch to fat metabolism mode – so don't push yourself or strain. These strategies can help keep your blood sugar balanced during the Colorado Cleanse:

❖ Be sure that you are taking *Sugar Destroyer* before each meal (page 58).

❖ Read and follow *Eat 3 Meals a Day – No Snacking* on page 67 or my book *The 3-Season Diet*.

❖ Add lean protein with lunch when the digestive fire is strong – or with all meals if needed. You can mix a nonfat protein powder, such as whey, rice or vegetable protein powder, into water or nonfat nondairy milk, such as rice milk. If you eat meat, you can eat lean chicken.

Q: What are the symptoms of unstable blood sugar?

A: A simple test for checking your blood sugar, other than a blood test, is to see if you can comfortably make it through the day with only three meals a day. If you can do this without a craving, mood swings, need for a nap or a snack, then the blood sugar is likely okay.

Q: May raw agave nectar be substituted for raw honey?
A: No, it has a very high concentrated fructose content due to processing. Raw honey facilitates fat metabolism, is a natural detoxifying agent, and stabilizes blood sugar. It does not burn like a sugar.

Q: I am near vegan, so I wouldn't mind taking whey protein, but is there an alternative like beans or something else to stabilize blood sugar?
A: Yes, rice and beans are a perfect protein and are my first choice. Whey protein is only for those who have unstable blood sugar and still need to cleanse. Seeds which are on the list are also great. You can also try hemp, rice or pea protein powders.

General Questions

Q: I am nauseated and having loose stools today. I think it might be the herbs. What else can I do to ease my discomfort?
A: Cut back on the *Liver Repair* so to only 1 capsule a day. After a few days, add back 1 capsule at a time until you find the dose that is right for you.

Q: I've been getting heartburn lately, especially when drinking the hot water. Are heartburns part of the cleanse? Should I stop drinking the hot water?
A: Remember we are only sipping the hot water every 10-15 minutes (just 2-3 sips each time). Take 2 caps of *Cool Digest* before each meal.

Q: It would be helpful to know what possible detox reactions we might experience?
A: This is a tough question. As we are all so different I couldn't say what uncomfortable things to expect. Hopefully it is all good. Whatever we do experience is definitely a symptom of what may be an underlying imbalance. The problems we experience during the cleanse are VERY diagnostic and can be useful to treat an underlying problem that may have been hiding for years. Clearly the general stuff -- days of fatigue and irritability - are signs of cleansing. Many of us have gut and digestive problems that show up in the Main Cleanse and will be treated in the Post Cleanse.

SUMMARY
CLEANSE AT A GLANCE

General Cleansing Guidelines
Follow the General Cleansing Guidelines during the
2 week Colorado Cleanse and continue for 2 more weeks afterwards.

Do the best you can. We understand that life can be unpredictable.

Begin taking these herbs before meals on Day 1:
1. **Sugar Destroyer :** Take 1 cap, 3x/day 15 minutes before meals with 12oz of warm water.
2. **Warm Digest or Cool Digest**: Take 1 cap, 3x/day, 15 minutes before meals with 12oz of warm water.
3. **Beet Cleanse**: Take 1 cap, 3x/day, 15 minutes before meals with 12oz of warm water.

Begin taking these herbs after meals on Day 1:
4. **Manjistha:** Take 1 cap, 3x/day, after meals for 4 weeks. As it is a red root, like beets, it may turn urine a pinkish color – this is normal.
   Are you sensitive?: Take 1 cap, 2x/day with food for 6 weeks.
5. **Turmeric Plus**: Take 1 cap, 3x/day, after meals for 4 weeks total.
   Are you sensitive?: Take 1 cap, 2x/day with food for 6 weeks.
6. **Liver Repair**: Take 1 cap, 3x/day, after meals for 4 weeks.
   Are you sensitive?: If you experience loose stools or cramps, decrease to 1 cap after breakfast and lunch. If problem persists, take 1 cap after lunch only.
7. **Regenerate:** Take 1 cap, 3x/day, after meals for 4 weeks.

Continue these guidelines during the entire Colorado Cleanse:
1. Take the herbs above.
2. From the Gaiam DVD, *Ayurveda for Detox*, practice:
   * ❖ **Everyday Yoga***: 10-15 minutes, 1- 2x/day (or Sun Salutations on

page 139)
- ❖ **Breathing***: 5-10 minutes 1 – 2x/day after yoga
- ❖ **Breathing Meditation***: 10-20 minutes 1 – 2x/day after breathing
3. **Eat three meals a day**, with no snacks.
4. **Sip hot water** every 10-15 minutes.
5. **Drink ½ your ideal body weight in ounces** of water per day.
For instance, if you weigh 140 pounds, drink 70 oz per day.
If you weigh 220 pounds but your ideal body weight is 140 pounds, drink 70 oz per day.
6. Do the **short daily oil massage** (before, during or after your shower).*
7. **Avoid wheat, gluten, dairy, coffee, alcohol, oils, cold foods and sweeteners** (except raw honey – a small amount is okay).
Get your oils naturally from seeds, fruits and veggies.
8. **Avoid eggs, fish, nuts, shellfish and peanuts**.
9. **Perform nasal breathing exercise** whenever possible.*

Pre-Cleanse
(Days 1-4)

1. Continue all the *General Cleansing Guidelines* above.
2. Eat a low fat diet with rice, beans, soup, salad, seeds, fruit and vegetables.
3. Eat 1-2 raw beets a day (see Beet Tonic recipe on page 85) with a meal. Best Option: Use *Beet Cleanse* formula in addition to – or in replace of – eating the raw beets. You will receive the best results by doing both.
4. Drink 1-2 Green Smoothies a day (recipe on page 86) with a meal or as a meal replacement.
5. Drink 4 eight-ounce glasses of organic apple juice each day. Preferably fresh squeezed. One glass of juice can replace a glass of water.
6. Eat as many apples as you can.
7. Add whey protein or lean meat only if needed to stabilize blood sugar levels.

Main Cleanse
(Days 5 - 11)

1. Continue the *General Cleansing Guidelines* above.
2. Take the indicated dosages of warm, melted ghee first thing in the morning. (Not hot.) *Measure the ghee before melting it.*
3. Eat a NON fat diet of khichadi (see Meal Options). Preferably follow Option 1.
4. On the evening of Day 11, take 4-6 teaspoons of Castor Oil. Though castor oil is preferable, you can take 1 ½ cups of prune juice.
5. If you experience low blood sugar or fatigue, follow Meal Options 2, 3, or 4 to be comfortable during the Main Cleanse. (Pages 96)

Morning Ghee

- Day 5 : 2 tsp of ghee
- Day 6: 4 tsp of ghee
- Day 7: 4 tsp of ghee
- Day 8: 6 tsp of ghee
- Day 9: 8 tsp of ghee
- Day 10: 8 tsp of ghee
- Day 11 : 10 tsp of ghee

Post Cleanse
Reset Digestion (Days 12-14)

1. Continue all of the *General Cleansing Guidelines* above
2. Eat a LOW fat diet.
3. Eat rice, beans, soup, salad, seeds, fruits and vegetables (see Recipes).
4. You do *not* need to eat Beet Salad or Green Smoothies unless you enjoy them, but do continue taking the *Beet Cleanse* capsules.
5. Add whey protein or lean meat with meals, only if needed to stabilize blood sugar.

6. **Digestive Strength Protocol:** To reset the digestion, cleanse the bile, pancreatic ducts and biliary tubes in the liver follow the Digestive Strength Protocol below. *To make the lemon water, mix the juice of 1 lemon in 16 ounces of water:*

Day 12: Take 2 capsules of *Beet Cleanse* and *Warm Digest* or *Cool Digest* 15 minutes before each meal with 12 ounces of lemon water. Sip 4 more ounces of lemon water during the meal.

Day 13: Take 3 capsules of *Beet Cleanse* and *Warm Digest* or *Cool Digest* 15 minutes before each meal with 12 ounces of lemon water. Sip 4 more ounces of lemon water during the meal.

Day 14: Take 4 capsules of *Beet Cleanse* and *Warm Digest* or *Cool Digest* 15 minutes before each meal with 12 ounces of lemon water. Sip 4 more ounces of lemon water during the meal.

Day 15 – 19: For 5 more days, take 2 capsules of *Beet Cleanse* and *Warm Digest* or *Cool Digest* 15 minutes before meals with 12 ounces of lemon water.

Maintenance Diet
Follow for at Least One Month

For the next month, eat a normal diet with an emphasis on seasonally harvested foods. Please visit www.lifespa.com/grocery to see a grocery list and simple Ayurvedic tips for each season. Do you feel like you want to continue cleansing or have lost the desire for heavy food? Then eat a wheat-, dairy- and sugar-free diet.

Continue taking the herbal protocol outlined in the General Cleansing Guidelines.

PART II
PRE-CLEANSE
(DAYS 1 – 4)

The plan during the Pre-Cleanse is to initiate a natural burning of your fat cells. This will do two very important things: One is that when you are burning fat you lose your appetite, so the need and craving for bread, pasta and those rich, heavy, over satisfying foods will be reduced. Secondly, you are releasing fat soluble toxins and chemicals that may have been stored there for years.

Once you get into fat metabolism, the magic happens. These first couple of days are when the body puts up a small battle fighting against this notion that it is safe to burn the fat. If this happens and you start craving, just drink a big glass of water. In a study at Cornell University, ten minutes later, 80% of the cravings were gone. The hydration therapy we suggest includes sipping hot water *and* drinking one half your ideal body weight in ounces of water a day (for example if you weigh 150 pounds drink 75 ounces of water per day). Not only will this help curb cravings, these are lymph moving techniques and triggers that initiate fat metabolism.

So in these first few days of the Pre-Cleanse, our goal is to get you into that craving free calm state of fat metabolism. We are initiating a detoxifying chemistry in this Pre-Cleanse. No worries though: if for some reason you do not slip fully into fat metabolism in the Pre-Cleanse, you will in the Main Cleanse. Once you slip into fat metabolism you will feel calm, stable, and free of hunger - although you must stick with your three meals a day. Fat is a slow burning fuel so it allows you to have a long calm sense of endurance without the hunger, cravings or nervous anxiety.

CHAPTER 9
EAT A LOW FAT DIET

Low Fat, Whole Foods

Follow the General Cleansing Guidelines in Part 1, which are to avoid gluten, dairy, nuts, sugar and common allergens.

Eat a low fat, whole food, seasonal diet of rice, beans, soup, salad, fruit, vegetables and seeds (such as pumpkin, sunflower, chia, flax and hemp). Please see the recipe section on page 119.

Soups should be non dairy and low fat.

Avoid Oils
  ❖ Do not eat any oils, such as butter, olive oil, sunflower oil, etc.
  ❖ Oils from avocado or seeds are fine. You can eat rice cakes with avocado and salt.
  ❖ Salad dressing should be low in fat: raw honey and lemon, balsamic vinegar or other low or non fat dressings are fine.

Q: Are all oils out? Can I use a small amount of oil as long as I keep it lowfat during the Pre and Post Cleanse?

A: Please don't add any oil to anything during the Colorado Cleanse. Oil is concentrated and harder to digest. Small amounts of healthy, food based, unprocessed fat are okay during the Pre and Post Cleanse. For example, my favorite combo is rice crackers with avocado and a dash of natural salt. For breakfast I love freshly juiced apple, beet and carrot juice with raisins and some sunflower, pumpkin or hemp seeds. Nuts are too heavy during the Pre and Post Cleanse. So enjoy the low fat now because soon it will be mostly nonfat khichadi for breakfast, lunch and supper.

CHAPTER 10
EAT THESE 4 FOODS
TO THIN THE BILE AND FLUSH THE LIVER

These four foods will thin the bile and flush the liver, which will help escort toxins out of your body. You can eat these foods as part of your meals, or they can be the only thing you eat at a meal – or even perhaps the entire day. For example, you can have a Beet Salad Tonic with a cup of Green Soup for dinner. You do not need to eat them in addition to a typical meal, which can be too much food for most people.

While we are shooting for 3 meals a day, if you do find yourself experiencing cravings, then have a snack – preferably an apple. Try to make your meals bigger or with more protein the next day to help avoid the need for an in between meal snack.

Raw Beets

Eat 1-2 raw beets per day with meals. Beets are perhaps the best bile thinning agents. Beets can be juiced. Cooked or roasted beets are okay but raw is preferable.

Beet Salad Tonic
1 raw beet, peeled and grated
Juice of ½ a lemon
Dijon Mustard to taste (optional)
Combine all ingredients.

Options: for more flavor and variety you can add some fresh ginger root or fresh grated apple.

Q: After I eat the grated raw beet I feel good, then hours later if I eat anything else I feel nauseous and bloated on the left side, and the next morning I have really loose stools. Could this be a liver cleanse or should I stop eating the beets?

A: This is exactly that, a bile and liver flush. It is a good thing and I would continue. This kind of digestive nausea has to go and this should dissipate soon, by the end of the Pre-Cleanse.

Green "Soup" Smoothie

Drink 1 - 2 (8 ounce) glasses per day, as part of a meal. It is rejuvenating for the bile and liver. The following recipe is the most beneficial because steaming, then blending, helps break down the cell wall and releases vital nutrients.

Green Smoothie
3   stalks celery
2   whole zuchinni
2   cups of string beans
1   cup of parsley

1. Place 1 cup of water into a big pot.
2. Add the string beans, zucchini and celery to the pot. Steam them for about 8 minutes until tender but still crisp (don't overcook).
3. Put all the ingredients into a blender, including the fresh parsley and the water the vegetables were steamed in. Puree until smooth. You can add more water if needed.

Flavor Options:
- ❖ Sweet Smoothie: Add apple juice, an apple, ginger and/or lemon.
- ❖ Savory Soup: Add garlic and ginger with veggie broth to make it savory.
- ❖ You can use other greens on the seasonal grocery list.

In a pinch, green drinks from Odwalla or other sources will suffice.

Apple Juice

Drink 4 (8 ounce) glasses of organic apple juice each day. Dilute with water if you have blood sugar issues. Freshly juiced - rather than store bought - apple juice will be easier on the blood sugar and more effective if it is available.

Ideally, drink this *with meals* rather than making it a snack. However, if you are hungry in between meals drink some apple juice and at the next meal eat more protein so you don't have to snack again.

- ❖ You can mix a glass of apple juice into your green smoothie.
- ❖ You can add nonfat whey protein powder if you need extra protein.
- ❖ A glass of apple juice can replace a glass of water.

Q: I get gas when I drink apple juice with my meals. Isn't that bad food combining?
A: If you get gas from drinking apple juice with your meal this is an indication of a very weak digestive fire and sluggish bile flow. Apples will thin and flush the bile and are an important part of the Pre Cleanse. Do the best you can. In future cleanses this will become easier.

Apples

Eat as many apples as possible during the Pre Cleanse. You can eat them after each meal or as a snack between meals if you are craving anything. Apples help thin the bile and dilate the bile ducts and liver's biliary tubes which will be used for detoxification. Apple pectin is a great detoxifier for the villi and gut wall.

Q: I have candida and was told by my general practitioner to avoid fruits and veggies with high sugar content, such as beets and apples. What should I do instead?
A: Instead of the beets, you can have an extra glass of the Green Smoothie. Instead of apples and apple juice, you can enjoy more green drinks (such as celery, ginger, spinach, lime). You can also purchase coconut water from most health food stores - just make sure it is unsweetened.

PART III
SEVEN DAY MAIN CLEANSE
(DAYS 5 - 11)

Each morning during the Main Cleanse you will drink increasing amounts of melted ghee and eat a simple NONFAT diet of mainly khichadi. This will force your body into fat metabolism so you start turning over fat cells and releasing toxins. Because fat is a stable non-emergency fuel, you will feel calm when you enter fat metabolism mode. Fat is a detox fuel that will release molecules of emotion, fat-soluble toxins and 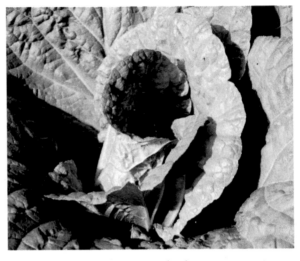 chemicals that are stored in our fat cells. Some of these include preservatives, DDT, dioxin, pollutants, pesticides and other cancer-causing chemicals.

Each morning the ghee will force the body into a fat metabolic state. The more ghee you take the more fat the body must burn. During the seven days of the Main Cleanse the golden rule is to eat a no fat diet. Without fat in the diet, the body will stay in fat metabolism all day. If a fatty food is eaten, the body will burn the dietary fat and stop burning body fat.

In this way the body slips in to a fasting state even though you are still eating three meals a day. Such a fast forces toxic fats to be released as well as fat soluble molecules of emotion. During these seven days the fat cells are emptied and fat, which is a stable and preferable fuel supply for the body, has replaced fast burning sugars.

The ghee also forces the gallbladder to flush toxic bile and clean the bile and pancreatic ducts. This allows the liver to be more willing to process stored toxins that are now in circulation.

The ghee also has a lubricating and calming influence on the soft tissues of the body and the nervous system.

A couple of reminders before we start:

Don't aim for perfection.

Be easy. This is not an endurance event.

Let the cleanse do its thing without strain.

If you are straining you are not burning fat.

Just do the best you can.

Remember there are food options so don't starve yourself.

Listen to your body.

Water helps with hunger pangs so stay hydrated.

Success Story
~ I feel energized and light and am able to stick to 3 meals a day, no problem. My husband was able to break his coffee/caffeine addiction. He experienced no headaches and has no cravings!! I lost 6 and my husband lost 10 pounds. Both of us feel so good! This is by far the best experience we've had cleansing at home. Thank you!

CHAPTER 11
MORNING GHEE PROTOCOL

Drinking ghee is not recommended if you have gallbladder trouble or difficulty digesting fat.

1. First thing each morning when you wake up, drink the prescribed amount of melted ghee. It is best to do this as early in the morning as possible on an empty stomach.
2. Melt the prescribed teaspoons of ghee and drink on an empty stomach.
3. Wait ½ hour before drinking or eating anything so that the ghee has time to collect toxins.

Morning Ghee

- Day 5 : 2   tsp of ghee
- Day 6:   4   tsp of ghee
- Day 7:   4   tsp of ghee
- Day 8:   6   tsp of ghee
- Day 9:   8   tsp of ghee
- Day 10: 8   tsp of ghee
- Day 11 : 10 tsp of ghee

Only increase the dose of ghee each day if you are tolerating it. If you experience loose, uncomfortable stools then do not increase the dose of ghee. Stay at the current dose until comfortable and then increase.

Special Tips

If it's difficult for you to drink plain melted ghee, add a ½ cup of warm soy, rice or almond milk. (Though we recommend avoiding soy during the Colorado Cleanse, it does cut the taste of the ghee the best). Warm the ghee and the "milk" to the same temperature so they mix easily and then drink it all at once. If needed, you can add a pinch of nutmeg, cinnamon and/or cardamom

Try holding your nose while sipping the ghee and rinsing the cup out.

Chase the ghee down with ½ a cup of ghee-free soy milk.

Use flax seed, coconut or olive oil if you prefer not to use ghee.

If nausea occurs, sip ½ - 1 cup of warm-to-hot water with fresh lemon juice and grated ginger root. Eat a little khichadi ½ hour after drinking the ghee even if you feel full. This helps settle the stomach.

Daily Guidelines

Continue taking medications.

It is best to stop taking supplements that are not part of the Colorado Cleanse - but take them if you feel you cannot do without them.

If you are taking fish oil or omega oils, discontinue them during the Main Cleanse. If you feel you cannot do without them, take them with the ghee in the morning.

Continue with all the *General Cleansing Guidelines* on pages 45-82 (herbs, daily yoga, meditation, breathing, self massage, etc.).

Advanced Ghee Cleanse

If you want to increase the benefits of the Main Cleanse, you can increase your dosage of ghee each morning using *Advanced Ghee Dosages* at right. You will need to ensure you have enough ghee on hand, which would be a total of 84 teaspoons of ghee (about 1 lb).

If you are uncomfortable at all, decrease to the regular dose or whatever dose is comfortable for you. This is not about enduring, suffering, or proving anything. If you are not feeling well with a higher dose of ghee it is because it isn't the right dose for you – it isn't because you are not tough enough.

Advanced Ghee Dosages

- Day 5 :   3   tsp of ghee
- Day 6:   6   tsp of ghee
- Day 7:   9   tsp of ghee
- Day 8:   12 tsp of ghee
- Day 9:   15 tsp of ghee
- Day 10:   18 tsp of ghee
- Day 11 : 21 tsp of ghee

Only increase the dose of ghee each day if you are tolerating it. If you experience uncomfortable loose stools then do not increase the dose of ghee. Stay at the current dose until comfortable and then increase.

Freqently Asked Questions About the Ghee

Q: Does ghee (a saturated fat) raise the LDL cholesterol and triglyceride levels?
A: This is a good question. Yes, ghee alone will raise your cholesterol if it is taken at high dosages for a long period of time. According to the Ayurvedic texts, ghee raises cholesterol much slower than any other vegetable oil. During the Colorado Cleanse we are eating a NON Fat diet and are only taking the ghee for seven days. During the cleanse, after taking the ghee each morning, the body is naturally forced into fat metabolism mode which not only removes the ghee from the body but the toxic fat soluble chemicals stored in the fat cells as well. Studies show that this process actually lowers cholesterol.[1]

Q: Why is ghee better than other oils - such as olive oil, coconut oil or sesame oil?
A: Ghee has unique properties and that is why it is the oleation oil of choice for so many thousands of years:
- ❖ It cools the body while strengthening the digestion.
- ❖ It reduces acidity in the digestion and in the tissues.
- ❖ It's light nature (low saturated fat content) makes it easily digested and allows the fatty acids to penetrate the deep tissues and deeply and thoroughly oleate the tissues.
- ❖ Ghee also acts a carrier for the nutrition to be carried across the gut wall and chelate toxins to be removed from the cells. Other oils are too heavy for this.

Q: How do I know if I'm having gall bladder problems? What are the sensations?
A: Gall bladder problems usually manifest with a sharp or dull pain under the right side of the rib cage. There is sometimes referred pain to the shoulder blade area in the mid back. This is also made worse by eating a fatty meal. We are provoking a gentle cleanse of the liver and gall bladder by taking the ghee. I would suggest that you reduce the ghee to the dose that did not cause this pain if this is happening for you.

Q. Why do we increase the dosage of ghee everyday and how does that work in the body?

A: Yes, good question. We slowly flush the gall bladder because this process can overwhelm the gall bladder if we give it too much ghee too soon. So we slowly exercised the gallbladder by flushing with higher doses of ghee each day. The last night is a big flush with ghee in the AM and castor oil in the PM as the final flush. I have some video newsletters about the need to flush the bile that may be helpful. Please see my free articles online:

❖ *Surprising Symptoms of Digestion* (www.lifespa.com/digestivehealth)
❖ *Look and Feel Vibrant in 3 Steps* (www.lifespa.com/skin)
❖ *The Miracle of Lymph* (www.lifespa.com/lymph)

Q: If I am menstruating should I make any adjustments to the cleanse?
A: You do not need to make any adjustments unless you are not feeling good and strong. In that case, during the Main Cleanse, you don't have to increase the ghee each day (per the instructions for tolerating the ghee). As always, listen to your body.

References
1. Alternative Therapies in Health and Medicine, Sep/Oct 2002, Maharishi University of Management, Dr Robert Herron and Dr John Fagan. The effects of Ayurveda Panchakarma therapy.

Success Story
~ Four weeks after the cleanse I am able to easily stick to three meals a day with no more mid afternoon sugar crash and cravings!

CHAPTER 12
LAXATIVE THERAPY ON THE EVENING OF DAY 11

The purpose of the laxative therapy is to cleanse the body of impurities which have been loosened by the ghee (oleation).

The laxative is an important step of the cleanse – do not skip it.

1. On the evening of Day 11, your evening meal should be very light.

2. Before taking the laxative, take a 15-20 minute hot bath to increase circulation and loosen the impurities. (If a bath is not possible, you may substitute a hot shower or rest with a hot water bottle on your lower abdomen.)

3. Take 4-6 teaspoons of castor oil or 1 ½ cups of prune juice. Castor oil is preferred and is included in the Colorado Cleanse Supply Kit). If you have a sensitive stomach or bowel irritation, take prune juice instead.

   Take 4 tsp of castor oil if you tend to have frequent or loose stools.

   Take 6 tsp of castor oil if you tend to have normal to constipated bowel function.

   Castor Oil Tip: Juice one orange and slice another one into quarters. Put castor oil in ½ cup warm water. Mix juice from one orange into the cup with the castor oil and stir vigorously. Hold nostrils and drink. Bite into the other orange for about 5 seconds. Rinse cup. Release nostrils.

4. You will likely feel a laxative effect in 1-15 hours (average time is about 4-6 hours). It is okay if you do not have a laxative effect.

Q: I have to work early/travel on day 12. Should I do the laxative on a different day?
A: If you have to wake up early the next morning and go somewhere, do the laxative earlier in the evening or do the laxative a day earlier or a day later. If you do it a day later, stick to the diet but you don't have to do the ghee that day.

Q: Is the laxative going to be very uncomfortable? What should I expect?
A: You will have 3-10 loose bowel movements. There may be some cramping in your belly, but you will feel lighter and cleaner. The ghee has moved toxins to your lymph, which has brought them to your digestion. The laxative will help clear all these toxins out. Some people do not have a laxative effect, which is okay - the castor oil is still purging toxins from your digestive tract.

Q. After the castor oil I had several bowel movements. I woke up feeling clear but also very dehydrated and dull. I'm thinking I should take some electrolytes?
A: Yes definitely you should take some electrolytes and some protein, as in Meal Option 4 on page 98, right away to stabilize.

Success Story
~ My husband and I tend to argue about the same things over and over again, which makes me depressed. So, having the mono-diet and reflecting has really strengthened my resolve to behave and react in more productive ways. Even with the emotional releases that are hard when they are happening, I am so happy with this cleanse and have been in wonderful spirits since.

CHAPTER 13
KHICHADI DURING THE MAIN CLEANSE

Khichadi is your new best friend during the Main Cleanse. It is ideal to eat nonfat khichadi exclusively for breakfast, lunch, and dinner. Khichadi pulls toxins from your body, is high in protein, balances blood sugar, is extremely easy to digest and healing to your digestive tract and intestinal mucosa.

Please note that only eating khichadi is not for everyone.

The main point is to eat a no fat diet.

Balanced blood sugar and comfort allow the nervous system to disarm and relax, which is key to a beneficial detox.

Choose a meal option below that will not cause stress or strain.

If you ordered the Colorado Cleanse Supply Kit, you received 10 packets of khichadi. To make them no fat, simply pour all the contents of the packet into a pot with water and cook for 20-30 minutes – like you would cook rice. Do *not* sauté the spices with oil or add any extra oil, nuts, avocado, etc. You can use your own spices and herbs instead of the spice packet. Please see the 'Flavor Options' on page 101.

If you did *not* order the Colorado Cleanse Supply Kit, you can make your own khichadi with white basmati rice and split yellow moong dal beans.   We have included the recipe in this book on page 100.

You can cook enough to last 2-3 days and eat as needed.

Khichadi Meal Options

Follow the Meal Option below that helps you feel satisfied and your blood sugar balanced. It is more important to do what is right for you rather than strictly 'follow the rules.'

Option 1: Most Cleansing Meal Plan
Khichadi Only
Requires Strong Digestion and Balanced Blood Sugar

To maximize your cleanse and reap the most benefits, eat *only* nonfat khichadi. This will be incredibly healing to your digestive tract and extremely detoxifying. When you eat a mono diet, your body can focus the energy that normally goes towards digestion to cleansing and healing other systems. It is like baby food because it is very simple, easy to digest and healing to the gut wall.

Always eat your largest serving of khichadi mid-day when your digestion is the strongest. Eat a light dinner early or sip some hot ginger or hibiscus tea.

On this meal plan you can eat 4 meals per day if needed to keep your blood sugar and energy stable.

Option 2: Cleansing Meal Plan A
Khichadi and Steamed Veggies
Requires Good Digestive Strength and Fairly Balanced Blood Sugar

If your blood sugar becomes unstable or eating only khichadi is uncomfortable, then add vegetables at lunch: steamed vegetables or vegetable soup in a light, nonfat vegetable broth.

Option 3: Cleansing Meal Plan B
Khichadi, Steamed Veggies, Fruit and Salad
Good for Weaker Digestion and Imbalanced Blood Sugar

If you need more than khichadi and steamed vegetables, you can add cooked fruit in the morning with nonfat cooked cereal (such as gluten-free steel cut oatmeal or cream of rice) and salad at lunch with a nonfat dressing. This plan is not as detoxifying as Option 1 and 2 above. Please keep in mind that salad is most appropriate in the warm days of summer and less appropriate in the cold winter months.

Option 4: Blood Sugar Balancing Plan
Khichadi, Steamed Veggies, Fruit, Salad and Lean Protein
Best for Weak Digestion and Blood Sugar Issues

If you find that your blood sugar is imbalanced or if you are bored out of your mind and psychologically absolutely cannot handle eating only khichadi, then do the Option 2 or 3 meal plan. If you still need more food or variety, or your blood sugar is still imbalanced, then you can supplement with the following foods. At no time during your cleanse do we want you to feel like you are starving or suffering as it is also important that your nervous system is calm. During future cleanses you can work your way up to Options 3, 2 and then 1.

Breakfast can be nonfat, cooked, whole grain cereal. The best option is gluten-free steel cut oatmeal or cream of rice.

- ❖ You can enjoy some seasonal, fresh, cooked fruit along with your breakfast if you'd like, such as cooked apples or pears. As well as some herbal tea, like hibiscus or ginger.
- ❖ Other options for breakfast are khichadi, egg whites with vegetables, or vegetable soup.

Lunch should be your biggest meal of the day. We want your body to feel nourished, so please, eat a BIG lunch. Options include:

- ❖ Rice with nonfat beans
- ❖ Nonfat vegetable soup (you can add beans)
- ❖ Salad with lemon/honey or other nonfat dressing

Dinner should be early and light. You can eat the same foods as lunch (above).

To stabilize your blood sugar: Increase the dose of *Sugar Destroyer, Beet Cleanse* and *Regenerate to 2 capsules each* before meals, and/or eat lean meat or drink nonfat whey protein in water with meals - as needed.

Frequently Asked Questions About Khichadi

Q: The khichadi packet says you can add vegetables but Colorado Cleanse guidelines say to just eat the khichadi. Can I eat vegetables as long as they are with khichadi?
A: During the Main Cleanse we generally recommend that you eat only khichadi unless you're noticing problems with low blood sugar. If that's the case then you can add some steamed veggies. Khichadi is very easy to digest though and will give you the greatest cleanse. However, it's important to keep your blood sugar stable, as well, so that your body doesn't feel stressed.

Q: I feel exhausted and fatigued during the Main Cleanse. Should O stop?
A: If you feel weak, dizzy or hungry on Meal Options 1, 2 or 3 add some lean chicken (or a nonfat whey protein drink) to your meals to bring your blood sugar into balance. Do not hesitate on this. If your blood sugar crashes it is uncomfortable and your body stops burning fat, which is where toxins are stored. Each time you do this cleanse your ability to use your fat as an energy source will improve, your blood sugar will balance and you will easily enjoy Meal Options 1, 2 or 3 during future cleanses.

Q: Can we substitute Brown Rice for White Rice in the Khichadi?
A: Brown rice is OK and I realize it has more nutrients. But the white basmati rice is actually quite nutritious and very easy to digest; brown rice requires more digestive fire to break down the husk. During the cleanse we are trying to take the stress off digestion and eat easy to digest food, baby food really, so we can heal and repair the gut during the main cleanse.

The Main Cleanse is only 7 days long.
A little discipline is good.
But if your blood sugar is low or you aren't feeling well,
please make adjustments so you stay strong and calm.

Recipes for the Main Cleanse (Days 5 – 11)
Ideally, eat only non fat Khichadi during the Main Cleanse.
We have included some additional recipes if you are feeling low blood sugar.

Khichadi Recipe
If you are using our khichadi packets with pre-mixed rice/beans/spices, please dry roast the spices and do not add ghee or oil as the packet recommends.
The recipe below makes enough for 3-4 meals. You can adjust the spices to your taste (many people like to double or triple the spices).

1   cup Split Yellow Moong Dal Beans* (see 'weak digestion' below)
½   cup white basmati rice
1   Tbsp fresh ginger root (add more if you like ginger)
½   tsp *(each)* turmeric powder, coriander powder, and cumin powder,
½   tsp *(each)* whole cumin seeds, brown or yellow mustard seeds
1   pinch hing (also called asafetida or asafoetida) *optional*
8   cups of water or vegetable broth
½   tsp salt (rock salt is best). You can add more if you wish.
1   small handful fresh chopped cilantro leaves

1. Wash split yellow moong beans (dal) and rice together until water runs clear.
2. Heat a large pot on medium heat and then add ginger root, turmeric, coriander powder, cumin powder, whole cumin seeds, mustard seeds, and hing. This dry-roasting will enhance the flavor. Stir all together for a few minutes. Be careful to avoid burning.
3. Add dal and rice and stir again so all the grains and beans are covered with the spices.
4. Add water and bring to a boil. Boil for 10 minutes.
5. Turn heat to low, cover pot and cook until dal and rice become soft (about 30-40 min)
6. The cilantro leaves and salt can be added just before serving.
7. Bragg's Liquid Aminos can be used to replace salt. Add after cooking.

* It's important to use SPLIT YELLOW MOONG DAL beans as they are easy to digest because the hard to digest husk falls off when split. Split yellow moong dal beans have cleansing qualities that pull toxins from the body. They are available at Asian or Indian grocery stores (be careful of yellow dye) or through LifeSpa. Different spellings include "mung" and/or "dahl". Do not use whole moong dal beans, which are green, or yellow split peas or lentils.

* For Weak Digestion, Gas or Bloating
Before starting to prepare the khichadi, soak the split yellow moong dal beans overnight. Drain and rinse before cooking.

Or, par boil the beans by covering with water and bringing to a boil. Drain and rinse. Repeat 2-3 times.

Flavor Options
Instead of using the spices in the recipe above, you can play around with your favorite blend of seasonings. It is best to stay away from anything spicy, such as Mexican, Southwest, Thai, Caribbean, or Cajun flavors. Adding vegetables or fruit turns it into Meal Options 2, 3 or 4.

Here are some ideas:
- ❖ Breakfast: make it delicious with cinnamon, raisins and nonfat rice milk.
- ❖ Prunes: cook pruned into the khichadi with a few cloves.
- ❖ Simple: salt and a squeeze of lemon juice.
- ❖ Refreshing Khichadi: salt, dill and fresh cilantro.
- ❖ Italian: add Italian seasoning and 2-5 Tbsp of tomato paste.
- ❖ 'Pasta' Khichadi: Make it plain with garlic powder, salt, and pepper.
- ❖ Khichadi 'Dessert': Make it plain with cooked pears.
- ❖ Cauliflower Khichadi: add roasted cauliflower and fat free salsa.

Rice Cooker Method
Nice and Easy! Follow the guidelines above for soaking or par boiling the beans. Dry roast the spices for best taste, then throw everything into your rice cooker for effortless khichadi! You can even travel with your rice cooker!

Recipes for Meal Options 2, 3 or 4
(To Balance Blood Sugar)

Feel free to be creative with your own recipes during the Main Cleanse.

Just keep in mind these main guidelines:

- ❖ Keep it NON-fat.
- ❖ Use vegetables that are in season and ideally cooked (not raw). Please see the current seasonal grocery list on pages 121-123.
- ❖ Though white basmati rice and split yellow moong dal beans are the most detoxifying, you can use your favorite whole grain and legumes (such as quinoa and lentils or millet and adzuki beans).
- ❖ Ensure that your meals are warm and moist or brothy (such as stews or soups).
- ❖ Use spices such as ginger, cumin, pepper and coriander to aid with digestion. Avoid spicy foods or flavors as our goal is to heal the intestinal villi.

Water-Sautéed Vegetables
1. Chop vegetables of choice and steam.
2. In a skillet, dry roast:
   ½ tsp cumin seeds
   ¼ tsp mustard seeds
   8 fenugreek seeds
3. Cover with lid and let seeds pop for a minute or two, then add ½ tsp cardamom.
4. Add vegetables, a ¼" of water, and water sauté approx 2-5 minutes until they are cooked to your desired texture. Keep the water boiling.
5. Salt to taste.

Split Yellow Moong Dal Soup

2 qts.	water
¼ - ½	cup split mung beans
¼	cup white basmati rice
¼	tsp cumin
1/8	tsp ginger
1/8	tsp allspice
¼ t	coriander
dash	pepper
Salt	to taste
1-3	Tbsp ghee
1-3	Tbsp love

1. Use any or all of the following vegetables: Chopped carrots, spinach, asparagus, or sweet potatoes.
2. Put everything in a big pot and simmer for 1-2 hours, or use a crock pot for 4-6 hours.
3. The soup is ready when the rice and dal are well-cooked and the soup has thickened somewhat.

Vegetable Soup

1. Chop 2-4 cups of spring vegetables and simmer in water.
2. In a skillet dry roast these spices:

1	tsp ground cumin
½	tsp mustard seeds
8	fenugreek seeds
½	tsp cardamom
1	pinch black pepper

3. Add spices to soup pot and cook approx for 1 hour.
4. Salt to taste.

Moong Dal
1. Cook the Beans:
   Simmer 4 parts water to 1 part split yellow moong dal beans for two hours. Be sure the dal is creamy and thoroughly cooked so it digests well.
2. Separately dry roast:
2	whole cloves
1	tsp cumin seeds
½	tsp mustard seeds
8	fenugreek seeds
3. Cover spices with a lid and let seeds pop for a minute or two.
4. Add to the spice mixture:
1/8	tsp ginger
½	tsp cardamom
5. Let spices cook slowly for approx 1 minute, then add to the dal.
6. Salt to taste.

Sweet Potato Yam Soup "Good and Vata-Pacifying"

4-5	medium sweet potatoes or yams
1-2	carrots
6-7	cups of water
1	bay leaf
	salt and white pepper to taste
	cardamom to taste

1. Peel and dice potatoes and carrots.
2. Cook them with the bay leaf in about 6-7 cups water until soft.
3. Puree potato/carrot mixture with the same water for proper soup consistency; return to pot. Add seasonings to taste.
4. Heat thoroughly.

CHAPTER 14
GENERAL GUIDELINES FOR THE MAIN CLEANSE

Quantity of Food

Eat according to your hunger, but somewhat less than usual (between ½ to ¾ of capacity).

Seasonal Grocery List

Follow the non fat Grocery List for the current season (listed at the beginning of the recipe section) if you are following Meal Options 2, 3, or 4. This grocery list is different than what we have on our website or what we may have sent to you earlier as all items that have fat, gluten or are allergenic have been removed. You can eat anything you want off of this list if you are unable to follow the khichadi only plan or need extra support - however, eat them at one of your meals, not as a snack in between.

Snacking

If you are feeling the need to snack during the Main Cleanse, then have an apple and work on making your meals more satisfying. Your digestion is the strongest at lunch time, and it can burn through the big meal. If you eat a meal with a lot of protein, it will give you enough fuel in your tank to make it to dinner without crashing and having cravings. That's the goal. Play around with how big of a lunch you need so you don't need to snack later. When only eating khichadi, it is okay to have a fourth meal before bed.

Sip Warm Water All Day

Sip warm water every 10-15 minutes throughout the day. Ideally, you will drink ½ of your ideal body weight in ounces of warm water each day. Warm water helps re-hydrate your tissues a lot faster than cold water, and it's crucial to stay hydrated during the Main Cleanse.

Ginger tea is beneficial for digestion, mobilizes toxins, and restores balance. You may drink decaffeinated herbal tea. All teas should be taken with meals.

Tips for Staying on the Cleanse

If you are traveling, working or will be away from your home kitchen for more than 4 hours, bring khichadi with you in a tupperware or thermos so you are not stranded somewhere and starving.

If you are at a restaurant or eating with people who are not cleansing, simply eat khichadi beforehand or bring it with you so that you are able to easily stay on the cleanse. You can let the wait person know ahead of time that you are on a special diet but will tip them as if you are ordering a full meal (we've never had a problem bringing khichadi to a restaurant).

Most restaurants will make a veggie plate with rice or a potato. If you are at a Mexican restaurant, ask for rice and beans and a salad (without any dairy, salad dressing or guacamole).

Bring a rice cooker to work to make fresh khichadi. An hour before lunchtime simply toss the contents of your khichadi packet and some water into the rice cooker and turn it on. You can stash it under your desk, in a break room, a closet, a supply room, or anywhere out of the way. Your coworkers may even want to join you on the cleanse because it will smell so delicious!

If you are eating a meal at a friend's house, simply bring some cooked khichadi with you. If you don't have any cooked khichadi, bring your rice cooker (above) and cook it fresh without inconveniencing your host at all.

Making Khichadi on the Road

A previous Colorado Cleanser offered these wonderful suggestions – thank you!

> *"Warm a thermos, then put the contents of your Ayurfoods khichadi packet, or your own khichadi mix into the thermos. Add boiling water, mix well and close the flask tightly. The thermos will retain the heat and your khichadi will cook that way. I've cooked rice, soaked lentils and vegetables this way. Your ingredients*

should be at least room temperature (not cold) when you put them in the thermos. You may want to do a trial run before you start traveling. Cooking times vary. If the packet says cook for 15 minutes, check your thermos after 30-45 minutes.

Another way to cook khichadi on the road is to use the hotel coffeemaker. Put your rice, mung and spices in the clean coffeepot, pour the hot water in and mix well and keep the warmer on until it is cooked. You may need to add some additional water while it cooks.

I usually travel with a thermos flask and a small electric water kettle. If you have the thermos in your carry on bag, it will need to be empty to get past the TSA security screening. I put my thermos in a clear plastic bag with the lid in the same bag but left off so that the TSA staff can see that it is empty. "

Emotions and Food
Opportunities for Self-Inquiry

For most of us, the Main Cleanse is a wonderful opportunity to notice how much we use food to cover up our emotions or uncover an underlying blood sugar imbalance by snacking. When eating a mono-diet of only khichadi or a nonfat diet, your body is forced to burn fat and you may begin to experience some emotional stress or irritability. During the Colorado Cleanse we are not only detoxifying physical fat soluble toxins, we are releasing everything stored in our fatty tissue which also includes molecules of emotion.

There is a fine line between your emotional distaste for khichadi and your blood sugar actually crashing. When feeling irritable around the meal suggestions during the cleanse be sure to follow our blood sugar recommendations first. Then, once the blood sugar is ruled out, the opportunity exists for a deep emotional transformation during the Colorado Cleanse.

Many of us have used food as an emotional crutch for many years. When a food is not tasty we become emotionally dissatisfied. This diet is a great opportunity to break the control food has over you.

For thousands of millenniums, humans have lived on mono-diets, and most people in the world still have very little variety and eat the same thing every day. When we return to a normal diet, we can be grateful that we have access to so many different delicious and fresh foods.

Remind yourself that this meal plan is very temporary and it won't be long before you can eat other foods. When we are mindful with each bowl of khichadi, there is nothing to resist. We aren't thinking about all the other bowls of khichadi we have eaten and how many more days we have to eat it – we are in the moment, eating this one bowl of khichadi and noticing all of its textures and tastes and smells. This is a great reminder for *any* "mundane" activity we resist!

>>> Learn More:
   ❖ Read my free article *The Psycho-Physiology of Stress* at
      www.lifespa.com/stress.

Success Story
~ Before this cleanse I was suffering from extreme perimenopause symptoms of anxiety at night. Now in the post cleanse I have not had any episodes ...I have no desire to ever do another "crash diet" again - not after knowing how good it feels to feel good. My thinking is clearer and I feel more balanced. I am excited about how great I will feel as I continue and regain my good health. Thank you!!!

CHAPTER 15
SELF-INQUIRY EXERCISES
(DAYS 5 – 11)

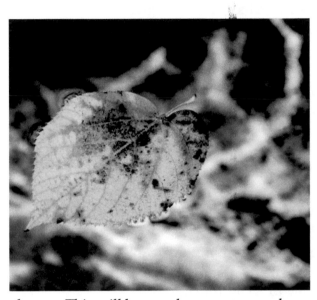

The Main Cleanse is a unique opportunity to release old emotional patterns that are stored in your fat cells. Not only will you be releasing physical toxins, you can transform old mental patterns, emotional beliefs, habits, and stress reactions.

So please find a journal and begin to document how you feel and what emotional issues or opportunities arise during the cleanse. This will be easy because as we cleanse we be begin to de-stress. We will become more sensitive and maybe a touch more irritable. So when that happens, try and see the emotional constriction as an opportunity to respond to that affliction with affection.

>>> Learn More:
   ❖ Read my free article *Detox Old Emotions and Beliefs* at
     www.lifespa/emotions.

Day 5
What Expands You?

Please list all the things you love:
- ❖ The things that truly expand you. What brings you joy?
- ❖ Then ask yourself: Am I doing these things?
- ❖ Then ask: If I am not doing these things, what is keeping me from doing the things I love?

List three qualities you love about your spouse, partner or loved one. Find a way to express your appreciation for these qualities throughout the day.

Day 6
What Contracts You?

Please list all the things that contract you. Opposite to what expands you, these are the things you do *not* love.
- ❖ They can be situations like public speaking, or people like your uncle Fred who is the most selfish, manipulating, intimidating person you know and you never know how to act around him.
- ❖ Make a list of the people that make you become a less desirable person.
- ❖ List the people with whom you have trouble being your most true, loving self when you are around them.
- ❖ List those people who provoke you and with whom you enter a conversation with your guard up and your weapons ready.

Pick one of the top offenders on that list and write them a love letter, including the things you love or appreciate about them. How did you feel when you wrote that love letter? Write down that feeling as well.

Day 7
Act with Love

Now that you have written a love or appreciation letter (or two), we are ready for the next step. I realize that writing these letters may have been tough. But if you have surrendered to this process you may have noticed that letting yourself love them was letting yourself experience the truth of the relationship. Let this letter become the template of truth, reflecting what is true about the relationship. Lets take action! Now is the time to use this letter for a model of how you interact with this person. Random acts of love and kindness can be expressed in an email, a note or a quick call of how you really feel. Let yourself express what you wrote in that letter. As you do this you will be breaking old mindsets that have convinced you that you cannot be your wonderful loving self because that person is unsafe, not nice or unworthy of your love. The reality is that when we hold back our true nature, we lose.

Day 8
Drop Childhood Personality Traits

Make a list of what personality traits you had to create as a young child to be safe and secure as your grew up. Who did you have to become?

Then ask yourself, what aspects of that personality are still serving you today as an adult and what aspects of your personality are not? Which aspects of your personality are holding you back?

Ask yourself, what would you lose if you dropped those personality traits?

Day 9
Take a Risk to Be Joyful and Loving

I know this cleanse can bring up some emotional stress. If you have been irritable or emotional, then please review my past self inquiry exercises to break some old emotional patterns. These patterns rear their ugly heads when we are stressed and while we are detoxing old fat cells. We are here. So please go for it.

By now you may be realizing more about some of your personality traits. You may begin to see that most of what irritates you is a choice. We often try to make others wrong and ourselves right to feel safe. Write down how it feels to be right, and how it feels to make someone wrong. You may notice that being right isn't as good as it seems.

In addition, it is time to create action steps. To move through and expose these behavior traits as the illusions they are. If you are afraid of someone or something, create a plan to let yourself be free to interact with them as your open, free and loving self. Make an effort to express affection where you would usually not. It doesn't have to be big, just a subtle way of letting your joy out. Remember, it is your joy and your life. Why should we let anyone keep us from experiencing the most precious part of ourselves?

Take a risk to be joyful and loving!

Day 10
Your Emotional Foot Print

Ever wonder what your emotional foot print is like? It is like when you walk through a garden, do the plants expand and reach out to greet you or do they contract and reel out of your way? Do we even know that how we walk through the garden makes an impression on our environment? This is our emotional footprint.

In life we often wonder why someone is acting mean to us and we figure they are having a bad day and either let it go or react to their anger. Consider this: perhaps a day or two ago you were making fun of that person or being critical of them, or somehow being passively aggressive toward them. Perhaps you hurt them without realizing it. This is your emotional footprint. What you are experiencing today may be the result of your unconscious actions yesterday. Be careful how you walk through the garden because each step may literally come back at you!

PART IV
POST-CLEANSE: RESET DIGESTION
(DAYS 12 – 14)

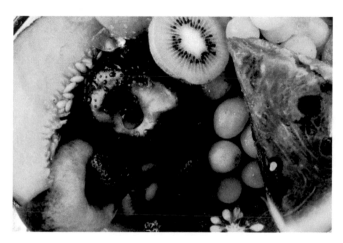

While this last phase of the Colorado Cleanse should be easy and a pleasant relief, it may be one of the most important phases of the cleanse to do well.

So often we do a detox or fast and then when we break it, go nuts and ravenously eat everything under the sun. In the Colorado Cleanse we are going to take these next three days to prepare the body to re-enter into a normal diet. We are going to turn the eliminative function and digestive fire back on so that when we do go back to eating seasonal foods we are ready to digest, assimilate and detox ourselves fully.

CHAPTER 16
POST CLEANSE GUIDELINES

Continue following the *General Cleansing Guidelines*.

Water: Continue sipping hot water *and* drinking one half your ideal body weight in ounces of water per day. This is very important now as we turn the digestive fire back on. Water protects the stomach lining so it can permit the increase of stomach acid production.

Yoga, Breathing and Meditation: Please continue to incorporate this into your daily routine. In the days and weeks after the cleanse we are much more able to develop long term flexibility so please take advantage of this opportunity now.

Follow the Digestive Strength Protocol on page 116.

Dietary Guidelines - Same as the Pre-Cleanse

Eat a low fat diet of rice, beans, soup, salad, seeds, fruits, and vegetables.

Enjoy fruit and fresh squeezed fruit and vegetable juices.

Eat as many salads and steamed veggies as you like. Eat more cooked vegetables than raw foods in the winter.

Rice, beans, oatmeal and potatoes will help make each meal satisfying.

Add seeds for healthy fat and protein.

Avoid nuts as they are heavy and harder to digest.

You do not have to eat raw beets or the Green Smoothie, but please continue if you like them.

Do not add any sugar, oils, wheat or dairy to the diet.

Soups should be non dairy and low fat.

Salad dressing should be low in fat – raw honey and lemon, balsamic vinegar or other low or no fat dressings will be fine.

Keep your blood sugar balanced. See pages 58, 67 and 77 for guidelines.

Improve Digestive Strength

After the Main Cleanse, we will reset your upper digestive strength, which is the most common cause of digestive distress.   Due to stress, intestinal inflammation, sluggish bile flow, dehydration and congestion in the liver, the digestive acids in the stomach can become reduced. When bile flow is congested and slow, it is not able to neutralize the stomach acids. The body attempts to temporarily solve the danger of high acids entering the small intestine by reducing acid production in the stomach, which leads to digestive weakness, the need for supplemental enzymes, poor assimilation of nutrients and the accumulation of undigested food, which can be toxic. Without proper digestive strength in the stomach, the entire digestive process is compromised.

Many people find themselves adjusting their diets to accommodate such weakened digestion by avoiding wheat, dairy, soy, fat, fried food, heavy food or by eating more veggies. While it is healthy to eat a clean diet, if we are doing it because we feel sick otherwise then we are eating healthy for the wrong reasons. Now that we have thinned healed the gut, the bile and lymph, and detoxed the body we are ready to turn the digestive fire back on.

>>> Learn More:
   ❖ Free Health Report and Video: *Surprising Symptoms Linked to Poor Digestion* at www.lifespa.com/digestivehealth.

Digestive Strength Protocol

To reset the digestion, follow the below Digestive Strength Protocol during Days 12-19. *To make the lemon water, mix the juice of 1 lemon in 8 ounces of water.*

Day 12: Take 2 capsules of *Beet Cleanse* and *Warm Digest* or *Cool Digest,* 15 minutes before each meal, with 12 ounces of lemon water. Sip 4 more ounces of lemon water during the meal.

Day 13: Take 3 capsules of *Beet Cleanse* and *Warm Digest* or *Cool Digest,* 15 minutes before each meal, with 12 ounces of lemon water. Sip 4 more ounces of lemon water during the meal.

Day 14: Take 4 capsules of *Beet Cleanse* and *Warm Digest* or *Cool Digest,* 15 minutes before each meal, with 12 ounces of lemon water. Sip 4 more ounces of lemon water during the meal.

Days 15 - 19: Take 2 capsules of *Beet Cleanse* and *Warm Digest* or *Cool Digest,* 15 minutes before each meal, with 12 ounces of lemon water. Sip 4 more ounces of lemon water during the meal.

Alternatives to *Beet Cleanse* and *Warm Digest* or *Cool Digest* :
- ❖ Alternatives to *Beet Cleanse:* 15 minutes before each meal and during and after each meal, drink ginger and/or fenugreek tea.
- ❖ Alternative to *Warm Digest:* Eat increasing numbers of 'ginger pizzas' before each meal (recipe on page 62).
- ❖ Alternative to *Cool Digest:* Add a pinch of ginger, cumin and fennel powder to hot water. Drink with each meal.

Q: I sometimes have acid reflux or heartburn which must mean I have too much digestive fire. Won't turning it back on make these symptoms worse? A: Actually studies show that the number one cause of heartburn is actually too little digestive acid, a disease called hypochlorhydria, so it is really important to understand the cause.

CHAPTER 17
FOLLOW THE SEASONAL DIET FOR ONE MONTH

For the next month, eat a normal diet with an emphasis on seasonally harvested foods. See pages 121-123 for seasonal grocery lists.

For best results, eat a wheat-, dairy- and sugar-free diet. This will allow the villi to totally heal and the digestive fire to be fully rekindled.

Q: Can you provide guidelines or tips for how to ease back into "normal" eating? I worry that I will completely fall prey to cake, cookies, ice cream, etc. after a restrictive diet. It seems that once I allow myself a small treat, I quickly fall into a sugar trap & want it all the time!

A: The nice part of the Colorado Cleanse is that the re-entry is built into the cleanse. In the Post Cleanse we reset the digestive fire so that you can digest and break down more difficult foods and thus will assimilate better and be more satisfied from eating healthier food and not feel that need to binge. Most cleanses starve you, and don't strengthen your digestion and assimilation so we are left hungry and dangerous!

Q: I'm surprised by how quickly I feel bad with the few times I've "cheated" on this cleanse. Why is that? I would hate to think that the only way to be healthy is to have a restricted diet forever.

A: The last thing this cleanse sets out to do is to leave you on a restricted diet. The goal is to prepare the body to detox normally by resetting good digestive function. The post cleanse is all about making sure we re-enter into normal foods by using the *Warm Digest* or *Cool Digest* to strengthen the digestive fire.

The reason you may feel bad when you cheat is because the khichadi is designed to heal and repair the villi. During this process the villi become very vulnerable and exposed. When you eat something off of the diet after eating khichadi for a few days your stomach will hurt. In India they call khichadi "baby food" because it is so gentle on the digestion. So when you have a milk shake or french fries it will irritate the villi that have just been cleansed and healed.

Q: If we are in situations (traveling, vacation, visiting people) where we cannot keep to the current seasonal diet during the coming weeks, is it devastating to eat some other foods once in awhile? And then return to the current seasonal diet as soon as possible?
A: No it will not be devastating at all, though I would suggest continuing with the current seasonal diet as much as possible in order to allow the villi to heal. Also, be sure to take the *Warm Digest* or *Cool Digest* before a large heavy meal so that it is broken down well and not an irritant to the gut.

>>> Learn More:

❖ Read my books *The 3-Season Diet* (www.lifespa.com/3seasondiet) and *The Yoga Body Diet* (www.lifespa.com/yogabody), which provide more information about transitioning to three meals a day without snacks, eating with the seasons, and recipe ideas.

Success Story

~ My digestion has improved immensely since I started the first cleanse, and it continues to get better even in the days after the fall cleanse. My digestion has been horrific for as long as I can remember, so this is a REALLY big deal! YAY!

RESOURCES

CHAPTER 18
RECIPES FOR THE PRE- AND POST-CLEANSE
Days 1 – 4 and Days 12 - 14

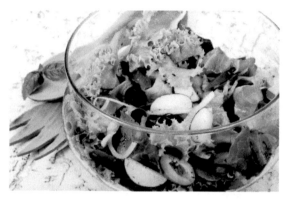

These recipes will help you immediately enjoy nourishing and delicious meals that meet the cleansing guidelines. Please share any of your favorites with fellow cleansers in our Online Forum. The recipes are divided into two categories: Spring/Summer and Fall/Winter. Please eat according to the current season for optimal results.

**Be creative and have fun with these new recipes.
Make up your own recipes based on the
dietary guidelines and Seasonal Grocery Lists.
Your meals can still be delicious even while cleansing!**

How to Water Sauté
Instead of sautéing vegetables in oil, water sauté them by bringing a small amount of water to a fast boil in a saucepan. Add small amounts of water as needed until the vegetables are soft.

Pureed Vegetable Soups
You can make vegetable soups by steaming your favorite vegetables and then blending them with veggie broth or unsweetened rice milk in a blender. Add spices such as lemon, seeds (for protein and creaminess), ginger, salt, pepper.

Carrot Soup: Steamed carrots with veggie broth, seeds (such as hemp), ginger, salt, pepper and cumin.

Spinach Soup: Steamed or raw spinach blended with unsweetened rice milk, seeds (such as sunflower), ½ an apple, salt, pepper and a dash of lemon juice.

How to Enjoy Greens

Spring and fall is the time to savor salads, micro-greens, sprouts and leaf vegetables such as chard, dandelion, kale, and spinach. Enjoy them raw, steamed or water-sautéed.

Many people find greens more palatable when they parboil them for 2-5 minutes in a shallow pan of water, then strain them. (This removes the bitter tasting compounds. If you drink that green broth it is surprisingly sweet and buttery).

Lemon juice and dried raisins or cranberries help the greens taste less bitter.

Collards make a great replacement for tortillas – simply add some rice and beans (or filling of your choice) with sprouts inside a collard leaf and enjoy like a wrap! You can keep the collard wrap raw or steam it briefly.

When you steam greens for 8-10 minutes and blend them into a soup-smoothie it allows the micro nutrients (minerals and vitamins) to become more bio-available.

Success Story
~ The foods are not hard to prepare and I feel like I could go on eating like this forever! It actually makes meal prep more simple and I love eating close to the source! I am grateful to find something that has "stuck" for me and will be part of my routine from now on.

Spring Grocery List for the Pre and Post Cleanse (March – June)

- ❖ **This list has been edited to remove all foods with fat.**
  For the full list see www.lifespa.com/grocery.
- ❖ Though these are not the only items you can eat, they are the most beneficial foods for this season.
- ❖ *An asterisk means it is best to eat more of this food.*

VEGETABLES	VEGETABLES	SPICES	LEGUMES	HERB TEA
*Alfalfa Sprouts	*Radishes	Anise	*All Sprouted	Alfalfa
Artichokes	Seaweed	Asafoetida	Beans	*Cardamom
*Asparagus	Snow Peas	Basil	Adzuki	*Chicory
*Bean Sprouts	*Spinach	Bay Leaf	Black Gram	*Cinnamon
Beets	*Swiss Chard	*Black Pepper	Garbanzo	*Cloves
*Bell Peppers	*Turnips	Chamomile	Fava	*Dandelion
*Bitter Melon	*Watercress	Caraway	*Goya	*Ginger
Broccoli		Cardamom	*Kidney	*Hibiscus
*Brussels Sprouts		*Cayenne	*Lentils	*Orange Peel
*Cabbage	**FRUIT**	Cinnamon	*Lima	*Strawberry Leaf
*Carrots	Apples	*Clove	*Mung	
*Cauliflower	Blueberries	Coriander	Split Pea	**DAIRY**
*Celery	*Dried Fruit (all)	Cumin		*Only Nonfat*
*Chicory	Grapefruit	Dill	**LEAN MEAT & FISH**	Nonfat yoghurt)
*Chilies, dried	Lemons, Limes	Fennel	*Lean meat only to*	(moderation)
Cilantro	Papayas	Fenugreek	*stabilize blood sugar.*	Rice/Soy milk, nonfat
*Collard Greens	Pears	Garlic	Chicken	*Goat milk, nonfat
*Corn	Pomegranates (sour)	Ginger	Duck (moderation)	
*Dandelion	Raspberries	Horseradish	Eggs (moderation)	**BEVERAGES**
*Endive	Strawberries	Marjoram	Freshwater fish	Black Tea
Fennel	All Berries	Mustard	Lamb (moderation)	(moderation)
*Garlic		Nutmeg	Ocean fish	Water
Ginger		Oregano	(moderation)	(room temp - hot)
*Green Beans	**GRAINS**	Peppermint	Turkey	
*Hot Peppers	Amaranth	Poppy Seeds		
Jicama	Barley	Rosemary	**SEEDS**	**SWEETENERS**
*Kale	Buckwheat	Saffron	Chia	*Honey - Raw
Leeks	Corn	Sage	Flax	Maple Syrup
*Lettuce	Millet	Spearmint	Hemp	Molasses
*Mushrooms	Oats, dry	Thyme	Pumpkin	
*Mustard Greens	Quinoa	Turmeric	Sunflower	**CONDIMENTS**
*Onions	Brown rice, long grain			Carob
*Parsley	Rye			Pickles
*Peas				
*Potatoes, baked				

Summer Grocery List for the Pre and Post Cleanse (July – Oct)

❖ **This list has been edited to remove all foods with fat.**
  For the full list see www.lifespa.com/grocery.

❖ Though these are not the only items you can eat, they are the most
  beneficial foods for this season.

❖ *An asterisk means it is best to eat more of this food.*

VEGETABLES	VEGETABLES	LEGUMES	BEVERAGES
Alfalfa Sprouts	*Squash, Acorn	*Adzuki	Water
*Artichokes	Squash, Winter	Bean Sprouts	(room temp or cool)
*Asparagus	Sweet Potatoes	*Black Gram	
Bean Sprouts	Swiss Chard	*Fava	**HERB TEA**
*Beet greens	Tomatoes (sweet)	*Garbanzo	*Chicory
*Bell Peppers	Turnip Greens	Goya	*Dandelion
*Bitter Melon	*Watercress	Kidney	*Hibiscus
*Broccoli	*Zucchini	Lentils	*Mint
*Cabbage	**FRUIT**	Lima	
*Cauliflower	*Apples	*Mungs	**SWEETENERS**
*Celery	*Apricots	*Split Pea	Maple Syrup
Chicory	*Blueberries	*Tofu	(small amounts)
*Cilantro	*Cantaloupe		Rice Syrup
Collard Greens	*Cherries (ripe)	**CONDIMENTS**	
Corn	*Cranberries	Carob	**DAIRY**
*Cucumbers	Dates		***Only Nonfat***
*Dandelion	Dried Fruit	**SPICES**	Cheese, nonfat
Eggplant	Figs	Anise	(moderation)
Endive	*Grapes	Asafoetida	Cottage Cheese, nonfat
*Fennel	*Guavas	*Chamomile	*Milk, nonfat
Green Beans	*Mangoes	*Coriander	*Rice/Soy Milk, nonfat
*Jicama	*Melon (all)	Cumin	
*Kale	Nectarines	Fennel	**MEATS**
*Lettuce	Oranges (sweet)	Peppermint	***Lean meat only to***
Mushrooms	Papayas (small amounts)	Saffron	***stabilize blood sugar.***
Mustard Greens	*Peaches (ripe, peeled)	Spearmint	Beef (moderation)
*Okra	*Pears		Chicken
Parsley	*Persimmons	**GRAINS**	Duck (moderation)
Peas	*Pineapple (sweet)	*Barley	Eggs (moderation)
Pumpkin	*Plums (ripe)	Oat	Freshwater Fish
*Radishes (moderation)	*Pomegranates (sour)	*Rice	Lamb (moderation)
*Seaweed	*Raspberries	Rye	Pork
*Snow Peas	*Strawberries	Wheat	Shrimp (moderation)
Spinach (moderation)	Tangerines (sweet)		Turkey

Winter Grocery List for the Pre and Post Cleanse (Nov–Feb)

❖ **This list has been edited to remove all foods with fat.**
   For the full list see www.lifespa.com/grocery.

❖ Though these are not the only items you can eat, they are the most beneficial foods for this season.

❖ *An asterisk means it is best to eat more of this food.*

VEGETABLES	FRUIT	SPICES	LEGUMES	BEVERAGES
Artichokes, hearts	Apples, cooked	*Anise	Mung – split, yellow	Alcohol
*Beets	Apricots	*Asafetida	Tofu	(moderation)
*Brussels Sprouts	*Bananas	*Basil		Black Tea
*Carrots	Blueberries	Bay Leaf	**DAIRY**	(moderation)
*Chilies	Cantaloupe,	*Black Pepper	*Only Nonfat*	Coffee (moderation)
Corn	with lemon	Caraway	*Buttermilk, nonfat	Water (warm or hot)
Fennel	Cherries	*Cardamom	*Cheese, nonfat	
Eggplant, cooked	Coconuts, ripe	Cayenne	*Cottage cheese,	**HERB TEAS**
*Garlic	Cranberries, cooked	Chamomile	nonfat	*Cardamom
Ginger	*Dates	*Cinnamon	*Kefir, nonfat	*Chamomile
Hot Peppers	*Figs	Clove	Milk, nonfat, not cold	*Cinnamon
Leeks	*Grapefruit	Coriander	Rice Milk, nonfat	*Cloves
Okra	*Grapes	*Cumin	Soy Milk, nonfat	*Ginger
Onions	Guava	Dill	Sour Cream, nonfat	*Orange Peel
Parsley	*Lemons	*Fennel	Yoghurt, nonfat	
Potatoes, mashed	*Limes	Fenugreek		**SWEETENERS**
*Pumpkins	*Mangoes	Garlic	**MEAT & FISH**	Honey - Raw
Seaweed, cooked	Nectarines	*Ginger	*Lean meat only to*	*Maple Syrup
Squash, Acorn	*Oranges	Horseradish	*stabilize blood sugar.*	*Molasses
*Squash, Winter	*Papayas	Marjoram	*Beef	*Rice Syrup
*Sweet Potatoes	Peaches	Mustard	*Chicken	Mint
*Tomatoes	Pears, ripe	Nutmeg	*Crabs	
Turnips	*Persimmons	Oregano	*Duck	**GRAINS**
	Pineapples	Peppermint	*Eggs	*Amaranth
	Plums	Poppy Seeds	*Freshwater fish	Buckwheat
	Strawberries	Rosemary	*Lamb	(moderation)
CONDIMENTS	*Tangerines	*Saffron	*Lobster	Millet (moderation)
Carob		Sage	*Ocean Fish	*Oats
Chocolate		Spearmint	*Oysters	*Quinoa
Pickles		Thyme	*Pork	Rice
*Salt		*Turmeric	*Shrimp	*Rice, Brown
Vinegar				Rye (moderation)
			*Turkey	*Wheat
			*Venison	

Fall/Winter Recipes for the Pre and Post Cleanse

Breakfast Inspirations

Enjoy some of these breakfast ideas. Be sure to eat enough to carry you through until lunch without getting too hungry or low blood sugar.

Tropical Fruit with Nuts and Rice Cakes
❖ Papaya and/or mango with chopped dates and sunflower seeds.
❖ Rice cakes with apple butter or yam butter.
❖ Hot herb tea (such as chamomile)

Burrito
❖ Burrito filled with split yellow moong dal chili (spice with turmeric, salt, ginger, cumin, cayenne and hing) with onions, corn, and tomatoes.) Enjoy wrapped in a raw or steamed collard or kale leaf.
❖ Rice cakes with avocado and sea salt.
❖ Hot Herb tea (such as ginger).

Hot Cereal: Lemon and Fig
❖ Cooked brown rice with ginger, slices of dried fig, pumpkin seeds, a pinch of cardamom and a few squeezes of lemon. Sweeten with a small amount of raw honey after cooking. You can cream the cooked rice in a blender before adding the toppings.
❖ Orange Juice (room temperature).
❖ Hot herb tea (such as spearmint).

Hot Cereal: Oats with Bananas and Coconut
❖ Cook oatmeal or oat groats with shredded coconut flakes. Add chopped dates, cinnamon, banana slices and hemp seeds.
❖ Fresh beet and carrot juice.
❖ Hot herb tea (such as ginger and lemon).

Hot Cereal: Apples and Millet
❖ Cook millet with sliced apples. Top with cinnamon, cloves, chopped dates, flax seeds and lowfat rice milk.
❖ Berry Basil Beverage: In a blender, lightly puree 1 cup of blueberries and strawberries with a handful of fresh basil leaves and juice of 1 lime in 1 cup of room temp water. Sweeten with raw honey if needed.
❖ Hot herb tea, such as a mix of orange peel, cinnamon and cloves.

Hot Cereal: Apricots with Amaranth
❖ Cook amaranth with cloves and fresh or dried apricots.
❖ Top with sesame seeds, a splash of lemon juice and lowfat rice milk.
❖ Hot herb tea, such as chamomile with orange peel.

Fall/Winter Lunch Inspirations for the Pre and Post Cleanse

To keep yourself energized and focused until dinner, eat a satisfying lunch between 10am – 2pm when your digestive strength is strongest. Do not eat with any distractions, such as TV, while working, reading, on the computer, or talking on the phone. Sit for a few minutes after you are finished before getting up from the table. Learn more at www.lifespa.com/meals.

Colorful Lunch
❖ Avocado-Tomato Salad (with artichoke hearts, fresh basil and lemon juice)
❖ Orange and Beet Soup (water sauté 2 celery stalks, 2 large carrots, 2 large potatoes, and 3 medium beets for a few minutes. Add 1 tsp salt and 1 cup orange juice and enough water to cover vegetables. Cook until tender. Add fresh black pepper and sea salt to taste.)
❖ Steamed okra, beets, or carrots or well-cooked broccoli topped with your favorite seed – pumpkin, sunflower or hemp.

Pumpkin Soup with Garlic Chard

❖ Pumpkin soup (sauté 1 large onion chopped and 4-5 cloves of finely chopped garlic until soft. Add 4 cups vegetable broth, 2 cups pureed cooked pumpkin **or** 1 cup canned pumpkin, 1 Tbsp seeded diced jalapeño, 5 medium red potatoes, diced into 1/2 inch cubes, 1 Tbsp oregano, pinch of cayenne or other red pepper, and 1/2 tsp cumin. Cook until potatoes are soft, about 30 minutes. Add 1/3 cup unsweetened rice milk, salt and garnish with pumpkin seeds, cilantro or parsley). If you want some protein, add pureed split yellow moong dal beans as a creamy – and protein rich – base.

❖ Steamed chard with water sautéed garlic, squeeze of lemon, and salt and pepper to taste.

❖ Rice cakes with avocado.

Yams and Quinoa

❖ Baked yam or squash (delicious plain or season with salt and pepper or cinnamon).

❖ Cooked quinoa (or millet or amaranth) with a few bay leaves, rosemary, sage, salt and pepper.

❖ Parboiled brussel sprouts with garlic, salt, pepper and lemon. Garnish with sunflower seeds.

Curried Dal and Aloo Mutter (Potatos with Peas)

❖ Split yellow mung bean soup (with tomatoes, turmeric, cumin, ginger, hing, coriander, salt, black pepper or cayenne)

❖ Aloo Mutter (Boil 3 potatoes, chopped, in water with 2 bay leaves until tender - about 20-25 minutes. Drain and set aside. Meanwhile water sauté 1/2 onion, sliced, in 1/3 cup water with, 1 tsp coriander, 1 tsp cumin, 1/2 tsp turmeric, 1/4 tsp ground cloves, and 1/4 tsp ginger. Add 1 cup peas and water sauté a few more minutes. Add potatoes. Garnish with lemon juice, salt and pepper)

❖ White basmati rice with a pinch of saffron and turmeric.

Miso Soup

❖ One pot quick miso soup: sauté garlic and ginger. Add a few cups of water and slices of carrots and beets. Parboil until cooked. Add cooked quinoa and miso paste to taste (always add miso after cooking to keep the enzymes alive.) Option: add wakame or dulse seaweed.

❖ Rice cake with avocado and sea salt

❖ Small green salad with (with lemon, salt, honey and garlic dressing).

Mexican Squash Mash

❖ Mash a cooked acorn or winter squash and blend in your favorite Mexican spice blend.

❖ Top with fresh corn kernels, thinly sliced red onion, sliced tomatoes and a few squeezes of lime juice.

❖ Small green salad with salt, lemon and honey dressing.

Potato, Leek and Fennel Soup

❖ Potato soup (water sauté sliced leeks and sliced fresh fennel until soft. Add veggie broth and diced potatoes. Simmer until very tender, about 25 minutes. Season with salt and pepper. Serve as is or puree.)

❖ Rice crackers

❖ Steamed kale with garlic, salt, pepper and lemon

Corn Chowder

❖ Corn and Quinoa Chowder (dry roast quinoa with cumin seeds and set aside. Water sauté fresh corn kernels, diced potato, and chopped onion for 5 minutes. Add veggie broth and lowfat unsweetened rice milk. Simmer until vegetables and quinoa are tender, about 15 minutes. Top with chunks of avocado and lime wedges.)

❖ Steamed asparagus with lemon

Fall/Winter Dinner Inspirations for the Pre and Post Cleanse

Enjoy an early and light dinner, ideally before 6pm. This will help you easily digest your dinner more easily and improve the quality of your sleep so you wake up more energized.

Squash Soup
❖ Acorn or winter squash soup (Cook cubed squash in veggie broth with onion, garlic, salt, and pepper. You can puree it until creamy if desired. This also tastes delicious with seaweed, such as wakame.)
❖ Rice cakes with apple butter.

Carrot Soup
❖ Carrot Soup (cook carrots in veggie broth with onion, potato, tomatoes and curry. Puree until creamy if desired.)
❖ Small green salad (with lemon, salt, and honey dressing).

Borscht
❖ Borscht soup (Cover sliced beets, cabbage and onions with 1 ½" of water. Bring to a boil and simmer on low until tender. Mash with a potato masher. Add a dash of apple cider vinegar and salt to taste.)
❖ Rice cakes with a thin layer of avocado.

Tomato Soup
❖ Tomato soup (puree tomatoes, ½ cup sun-dried tomatoes soaked in water – the dry kind, not the kind soaked in oil – with basil, oregano, rosemary, salt and pepper. Puree if desired. Garnish with sunflower seeds.)
❖ Rice cakes with a thin layer of miso paste.

Mung Bean Soup
❖ Mung Bean Soup (with carrots, potatoes, tomatoes, onions and curry. Add sea salt to taste after cooking.)
❖ Turnip-Apple Salad (chopped or grated baby turnips and apples tossed with lemon, salt, and honey).

Fall/Winter Side Dishes for the Pre and Post Cleanse

Enjoy these side dishes with your lunch or dinner meals. Paired with a green smoothie and beet salad they could be a complete meal.

Condiments for your Rice Cakes
- ❖ Cinnamon Yam Butter: Bake a yam and puree it with a pinch of cinnamon. Tastes delicious spread on rice cakes.
- ❖ A thin layer of miso paste (limit to 2 servings per week).
- ❖ Apple butter.
- ❖ Mexican Bean Pate (cooked split yellow moong beans pureed with garlic and your favorite Mexican spice blend).

Turnip-Apple Salad
- ❖ Chopped or grated baby turnips and apples tossed with lemon or apple cider vinegar, salt, and honey.

Tomato and Corn Salad
- ❖ Fresh corn kernels with diced tomate, thinly sliced red onion, fresh basil leaves, sea salt and black pepper.

Carrots with Orange Juice
- ❖ Water sauté sliced carrots in orange juice with grated ginger.

Sliced Turnips with Apple Butter
- ❖ Thickly slice raw turnips. Warm to room temperature. Dip in apple butter (or yam butter).

Fall/Winter Sweet Treats for the Pre and Post Cleanse

❖ Enjoy a sweet treat every other day (or less) only during the Pre and Post Cleanse, days 1 – 4 and days 12 – 14.

❖ Do not any sweets during the Main Cleanse.

❖ Refrain from eating *any* sweet treats during the Main Cleanse, days 5 - 11.

❖ Enjoy sweet treats with lunch (not with breakfast or dinner) when your digestion is strongest.

❖ Eat fruit at room temperature, rather than cold, because it is easier to digest.

Rice Pudding

❖ Cook 5 cups of rice milk with 1 cup of rice, 2 cinnamon sticks (or 1 tsp cinnamon), 1 bay leaf, 3 cloves, ¼ tsp salt, ½ tsp ground cardamom and 1 tsp vanilla extract. Sweeten with a bit of raw honey after cooking (our goal is to refine our taste buds so we enjoy the naturally sweet taste of rice). Top with chopped dates and sprinkle with rose water.

Pineapple with ginger

❖ Slice fresh pineapple and garnish with a few pieces of grated ginger

Tangerine Wedges with Blueberries

❖ Peel a tangerine and place wedges in a bowl. Garnish with blueberries.

Apple Crumble (or use plums, peaches or pears)

❖ Thinly slice apples with a mandolin or food processor (or by hand). Toss with lemon juice and fresh ginger and place in an oven safe dish. Cover with a crumble made of oats mixed with cardamom and cinnamon. Bake at 350 for 20-30 for minutes until apples are soft.

Mango Pudding (pure heaven!)

❖ Soak ½ cup dired mangoes in water for 30 minutes. Drain. Add to a food processor or high speed blender and puree until creamy with 1 ½ cups of chopped mango (or frozen mango thawed to room temperature).

Spring/Summer Recipes for the Pre and Post Cleanse

Breakfast Inspirations

Enjoy some of these breakfast ideas. Be sure to eat enough to carry you through until lunch without getting too hungry or low blood sugar.

Avocado and Rice Cakes
* ❖ Spread avocado and a dash of sea salt on your favorite rice cracker. Surprisingly good!

Grapefruit and Rice Cakes
From *The 3-Season Diet* by Dr. John Douillard
* ❖ Grapefruit with honey.
* ❖ Rice cakes with apple butter.
* ❖ Fresh carrot, beet and apple juice.

Southern Breakfast
From *The 3-Season Diet* by Dr. John Douillard
* ❖ Grits (cornmeal cereal with honey).
* ❖ Raw apples and pears (sliced with honey and cinnamon).
* ❖ Grapefruit with honey.
* ❖ Herbal tea.
* ❖ Fresh carrot juice.

Fruit Carpaccio
From *The Yoga Body Diet* by Dr. John Douillard and Kristen Dollard
* ❖ Grapefruit and strawberries slices drizzled with raw honey, ground cloves and a punch of freshly ground black pepper. Option: add pumpkin seeds for crunch and protein.
* ❖ Rice cakes with 1 Tbsp fruit-sweetened jam.

Rice Cream Cereal
From *The 3-Season Diet* by Dr. John Douillard
- ❖ Blend cooked rice in a blender with honey and a little rice milk. Garnish with choice of dried fruits, apples or raisins. Option: add seeds of your choice (pumpkin, sunflower, hemp or flax).
- ❖ Fresh grapefruit juice.

Oatmeal with Ginger and Berries
- ❖ Cook oat groats or oatmeal with rice milk, fresh ginger and cardamom. Garnish with a 1 tsp of raw honey and seeds of your choice (pumpkin, sunflower, hemp, chia or flax).

Millet with Dried Cranberries
- ❖ Toast millet in a medium saucepan at medium heat for 3-5 minutes. Add rice milk (2 cups of rice milk – or water - for each cup of millet) with cinnamon. Cook as you would rice. Add dried cranberries or raisins and seeds of your choice (pumpkin, sunflower, hemp or flax).

Spring/Summer Lunch Inspirations for the Pre and Post Cleanse

To keep yourself energized and focused until dinner, eat a satisfying lunch between 10am – 2pm when your digestive strength is strongest. Do not eat with any distractions, such as TV, while working, reading, on the computer, or talking on the phone. Sit for a few minutes after you are finished before getting up from the table. Learn more at www.lifespa.com/meals.

Salad, Rice and Beans
Rice and Beans: Cook your favorite rice with your favorite beans and spices. Choose from these legumes: adzuki, garbanzo, fava, goya, kidney, lentils, lima, mung and split pea:
- ❖ Adzuki beans with millet, ginger, miso and ume plum vinegar or brown rice vinegar.
- ❖ Lentils with quinoa and curry.

❖ Lentils or mung beans with brown basmati rice, Italian herbs and garlic.
❖ Kidney beans with white basmati rice and Mexican or Cajun spices.
❖ Enjoy with a salad or steamed veggies with lemon and salt from the Spring Grocery List.

Veggie Soup, Beans/Chicken and Kale
From *The 3-Season Diet* by Dr. John Douillard
❖ Vegetable Soup (made with rice or quinoa, carrots, green beans, celery, dandelions, mushrooms and onions mixed in blender)
❖ Rice cracker with avocado and salt.
❖ Steamed Kale (with balsamic vinegar or lemon, salt, black pepper and garlic).
❖ Veg option: baked beans (with basmati rice and asparagus)
❖ NonVeg option (only if needed to stabilize blood sugar): Grilled chicken breast (skinless and boneless, marinated in ginger-tamari sauce and grilled).

Greens and More Greens
From *The 3-Season Diet* by Dr. John Douillard
❖ Mixed Green Salad (with papaya slices, lime, a pinch of salt)
❖ Sauteed mixed greens (made with dandelions, spinach and mustard greens, water-sauteed with garlic and onions)
❖ Veg option: Garbanzo bean casserole (made with cornmeal, carrots, onions, fresh corn, tomato sauce, cayenne, coriander and sage)
❖ Nonveg option (only if needed to stabilize blood sugar): Broiled fillet of sole (rubbed with a mix of ginger, cumin, cayenne, paprika, cinnamon, anise and turmeric and broiled)

Spinach Salad and Artichokes
From *The 3-Season Diet* by Dr. John Douillard
❖ Spinach Salad (made with sliced mushrooms and nonfat vinaigrette dressing)
❖ Steamed Artichoke (with oregano, basil, bay leaf and marjoram)

❖ Mixed Green Vegetables (steamed green beans, cabbage, and broccoli with marjoram and pureed turnips and carrots)
❖ Veg option: Indian Style Rice and Beans (long-grain brown rice and split moong beans with turmeric, ginger and black pepper)
❖ Nonveg option (only if needed to stabilize blood sugar): Fillet of sole or flounder (braised in light chicken broth, finely sliced leeks, and minced shallots)

Green Bean Salad and Black Bean Patties
Fom *The Yoga Body Diet* by Dr. John Douillard and Kristen Dollard
❖ Green Bean Salad (made with cooked green beans, orange juice, tomato paste, garlic, thyme, chili powder, salt, and black pepper. Garnish with fresh bell pepper and some minced red onion).
❖ Black Bean Patties
   ▪ 2 cloves garlic, cut in half
   ▪ ½ red onion, quartered
   ▪ 2 celery stalks, chopped
   ▪ 1 C mushrooms, such as cremini or white button
   ▪ 1 C spinach leaves
   ▪ 1 can (15oz) black beans, rinsed and drained
   ▪ ½ C chunky salsa
   ▪ 1/3 C rolled oats (not contaminated with wheat)
   ▪ 2 Tbsp ground flax seeds + ½ C water pureed
   ▪ ½ tsp salt
   ▪ ¼ tsp black pepper

1. Place garlic in a food processor and pulse until chopped.
2. Add onion, celery, mushrooms, spinach, beans and salsa, and pulse until a chunky mixture forms (2 to 3 pulses)
3. Add oats, flax seeds or egg whites, salt, and pepper, pulsing once or twice, until mixed. Add more oats if too liquidy.
4. Form the mixture into 4 equal patties.
5. Heat a large nonstick skillet over medium heat. Add the patties and cook 4 to 5 minutes per side, until lightly browned and warmed through.

Herbed Rice

From *The Yoga Body Diet* by Dr. John Douillard and Kristen Dollard

❖ White Basmati Rice cooked with vegetable broth, garlic, shallots or onion, chili flakes, asparagus and spinach. Garnish with salt, pepper and fresh basil leaves.

❖ Spinach Salad (with roasted sunflower seeds and currants or raisins, with nonfat raspberry vinaigrette dressing)

Spring/Summer Dinner Inspirations for the Pre and Post Cleanse

Enjoy an early and light dinner, ideally before 6pm. This will help you digest your dinner more easily and improve the quality of your sleep. You will also wake up more energized.

Split Pea Soup

From *The 3-Season Diet* by Dr. John Douillard

❖ Split Pea Soup (made with rice and carrots, celery, onions and garlic)

❖ Rice cracker with avocado and salt)

Cream of Spinach Soup

From *The 3-Season Diet* by Dr. John Douillard

❖ Cream of Spinach Soup (made with rice milk, ginger, paprika, black pepper, and cooked spinach, blended and cooled).

❖ Rice cracker with avocado and salt.

Chickpea Soup

From *The 3-Season Diet* by Dr. John Douillard

❖ Garbanzo Soup (made with pureed garbanzo beans and chopped asparagus, cumin, cayenne, garlic and coriander, then garnished with fresh cilantro and lemon.

❖ Chopped asparagus with fresh parsley and a squeeze of lemon.

❖ Rice Crackers with a thin layer of miso paste.

Szechuan Fried Rice

From *The Yoga Body Diet* by Dr. John Douillard and Kristen Dollard

❖ Scechuan Fried Rice (made with rice, sunflower oil, ginger, garlic, adzuki beans or chick peas, red chili pepper, shiitake mushrooms, peas, red bell pepper and spinach. Sauce: apple cider vinegar, raw honey, salt. Garnish with thinly sliced scallions.)

Personal Pizza

From *The Yoga Body Diet* by Dr. John Douillard and Kristen Dollard

❖ Spread 2 slices of rice cakes with tomato paste. Top with minced garlic, bell pepper, spinach and pineapple slices. Bake for 5 minutes. Sprinkle with salt and basil.

Cream of Broccoli Soup

From *The Yoga Body Diet* by Dr. John Douillard and Kristen Dollard

❖ Cook broccoli, leeks, thyme, rosemary, paprika, cayenne, black pepper, salt, vegetable broth, and rice milk (until broccoli is tender, about 8-20 minutes). In a blender or food processor, add broccoli mixture with cooked navy beans and puree until creamy smooth.

Spring/Summer Side Dishes for the Pre and Post Cleanse

Condiments for your Rice Cakes

❖ Cinnamon Yam Butter: Bake a yam and puree it with a pinch of cinnamon. Tastes delicious spread on rice cakes.

❖ A thin layer of miso paste (limit to 2 servings per week).

❖ Apple butter.

❖ Mexican Bean Pate (cooked split yellow moong beans pureed with garlic and your favorite Mexican spice blend).

❖ Cilantro Pesto: pumpkin seeds, lemon juice, salt, cilantro.

Emerald Apple Sauce
- ❖ 2 apples   cored and cut in quarters
- ❖ Ginger   ½" slice of fresh ginger root or ½ tsp dried ginger
- ❖ Cinnamon   ¼ - ½ tsp
- ❖ Parsley   Optional: a handful of fresh parsley (tastes surprisingly divine. Start with a small amount if you aren't sure. You can even go up to a whole cup – or more!).
- ❖ Lemon juice   1-2 Tbsp, to taste
1. In a food processor or Vita-Mix (on speed 4-5) process until chunky.
2. Lasts up to 2 days in the fridge

Carrot Salad
- ❖ Carrots   6 carrots, scrubbed clean or peeled
- ❖ Orange   juice of 1 orange
- ❖ Dried Fruit   handful of dried raisins or cranberries
- ❖ Seeds   small handful of pumpkin or sunflower seeds (do not add the seeds if you are eating this during the Main Cleanse Days 5-11 to maintain the non fat diet).
1. Grate carrots by hand or in a food processor.
2. Toss with juice of 1 orange, dried fruit (and seeds if not during the Main Cleanse).
3. Leftovers can be added into smoothies, sautéed with celery, added to the beet salad, or eaten as a condiment.

Spring/Summer Sweet Treats for the Pre and Post Cleanse

Enjoy a sweet treat every other day (or less) during the Pre- and Post- Cleanse, days 1 – 4 and days 12 – 14. Do not any sweets during the Main Cleanse.

Refrain from eating *any* sweet treats during the Main Cleanse, days 5 - 11. Enjoy sweet treats with lunch (not with breakfast or dinner) when your digestion is strongest.

Fruit is easiest to digest when eaten at room temperature, rather than cold.

Grilled Fruit

❖ Bring 5 strawberries (sliced), and 2 Tbsp water to boil in a sauce pan for 2 to 3 minutes. Set aside.

❖ Coat a grill or grill pan with nonstick spray, over high heat.

❖ Grill pineapple rings for 4 to 5 minutes per side, until grill marks appear and the fruit softens.

❖ Transfer to a platter and drizzle with strawberry sauce and garnish with mint leaves.

Papaya with Lime and Chili

❖ Halve a papaya and remove the seeds (you can actually eat a few spoonfuls of the pungent seeds as they are excellent for your digestion). Sprinkle with lime juice and a dash of chili powder.

Pears with Raspberry Sauce

❖ Puree fresh raspberries (if frozen, let thaw to room temperature) with a few dates in a blender or food processor. Dip sliced pears into this sauce for an easy "fondue."

Apples with Cinnamon

❖ Slice apples and toss with a dash of lemon juice and sprinkle with cinnamon.

Success Story
~ I was experiencing Lyme disease like symptoms over the summer (big here in the east) with achy joints and fatigue. All that has gone away and my arthritic toe is starting to regain much of its range of motion.

SUN SALUTATIONS

The 'sun salute' is a complete Ayurvedic exercise also known as *Surya Namaskara*. This series of postures simultaneously integrates the whole physiology including mind, body, and breath. It strengthens and stretches all the major muscle groups, lubricates the joints, conditions the spine, and massages the internal organs. Blood flow and circulation is increased throughout the body.

It is a cycle of 12 postures performed in a fluid sequence one right after another. Each motion should be synchronized with the breath. By moving smoothly into each pose, breathing fully and easily through the nostrils, holding a pose for a minimum of 3 seconds, each cycles take about 1 minute.

If you are new to yoga I highly recommend taking a few classes with an experienced teacher to ensure that you have the proper alignment. If in doubt, move slowly and be gentle with yourself and your ability. You do not need to do the poses perfectly to benefit.

During the Colorado Cleanse, perform Sun Salutations for a minimum of 12 minutes each day.

How to do Sun Salutations

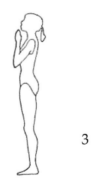
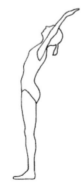
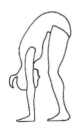

1. Salutation
Normal, restful breathing

2. Raised Arms
Inhale

3. Hand to Foot
Exhale

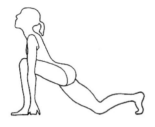

4. Equestrian

Inhale

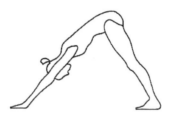

5. Mountain

Exhale

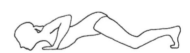
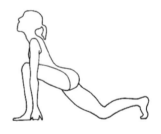

6. Eight Limbs

No breathing

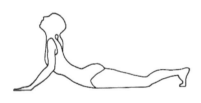

7. Cobra

Inhale

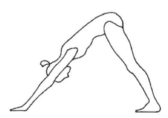

8. Mountain

Exhale

9. Equestrian

Inhale

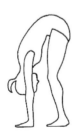

10. Hand to Foot

Exhale

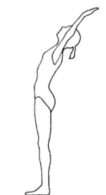

11. Raised Arms

Inhale

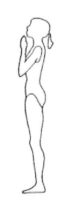

12. Salutation

Exhale

DAILY SELF-MASSAGE

The purpose of Ayurvedic daily oil massage, also called abhyanga is to assist in preventing the accumulation of physiological imbalances and to lubricate and promote flexibility of the muscles, tissues, and joints. The classical texts of Ayurveda also indicate that daily massage promotes softness and luster of the skin as well as youthfulness. The following are some simple instructions to assist you in learning the Ayurvedic daily oil massage.

Type of Oil

If you do not have the *Lymphatic Massage Oil*, use sesame oil. If you find sesame oil unsuitable in some way, you may also try olive oil or coconut oil. To purify the massage oil, "cure" it by healing it to about 220 degrees Fahrenheit, which is the boiling point of water. By adding a drop of water to the oil in the beginning, you will know that the proper temperature has been reached when the water boils. We suggest curing one quart or liter of oil at one time as this will cover about fifteen self-massages.

Note: As sesame and other oils are flammable, they should be cured:
 ❖ Always slowly heat oil on low heat, never on high heat.
 ❖ Oil should never be heated unattended.
 ❖ Once the oil reaches the proper temperature, remove it from the heat and store in a safe place to cool gradually.

Quick Self-Massage

Below are the complete instructions for a full Ayurvedic Daily Oil Massage. Ideally, about 10-20 minutes should be spent each morning on the massage. However, you do not have time, it is better to do a very brief massage than to skip it altogether – even just 1-2 minutes can bring you great benefit. In general, use circular strokes on the joints and long strokes on your limb, massaging towards the heart. You can do the self-massage while in the shower and the water is running over you – this keeps you warm, your pores open, and your skin hydrated. Once you have added this Daily Oil Massage into your daily routine, the benefits will naturally inspire you to continue.

How to Give Yourself a Complete Self-Massage

Heat ¼ cup of cured oil to slightly above body temperature. You can simply place your bottle of massage oil in a cup or bowl of warm water for a few minutes or heat it on the stove.

1. <u>Head Massage</u>: Start by massaging the head. Place a small amount of oil on the fingertips and palms and begin to massage the scalp vigorously. *The massage for the head and for the entire body should be with the open part of the hand rather than with the fingertips.* Since the head is said to be one of the most important parts to be emphasized during Ayurvedic Daily Self-Massage, spend proportionately more time on the head than you do on other parts of the body.

2. <u>Face and Ears</u>: Apply oil gently with the open part of the hand to your face and outer part of your ears.

3. <u>Neck</u>: Massage both the front and back of the neck, and the upper part of the spine. Continue to use your open hand, in a rubbing type of motion.

4. <u>Body Application</u>: You may want to now apply a small amount of oil to your entire body and then proceed with the massage to each area of the body. This lets the oil have the maximum amount of time in contact with the body.

5. <u>Arms, Hands and Fingers</u>: Next massage your arms. The proper motion is back and forth, over your long bones, and circular over your joints. Massage both arms, including the hands and fingers.

6. <u>Chest and Abdomen</u>: Now apply oil to the chest and abdomen. A very gentle circular motion should be used over your heart. Over the abdomen a gently circular motion should be used, following the bowel pattern from the right lower part of the abdomen, moving clockwise towards the left lower part of the abdomen.

7. <u>Back and Spine</u>: Massage the back and spine. There will be some area which you may have difficulty reaching.

8. <u>Legs</u>: Massage the legs. Like the arms, use a back and forth motion over the long bones and circular over the joints.

9. <u>Feet</u>: Lastly, massage the bottom of the feet. The feet are considered especially important, and *proportionately more time should be spent here* than on the other parts of the body. Use the open part of your hand and massage vigorously back and forth over the soles of the feet.

OVERWHELMED? HOW TO MAKE IT WORK FOR YOU

Are you new to eating this way?
Is your job physically demanding?
Does your blood sugar keep crashing?
Are you the only one cleansing in your family?
Are you travelling or ridiculously busy?

If the guidelines in this cleanse feel overwhelming, take a deep breath and be gentle on yourself. It is okay if you don't follow everything perfectly. Sometimes it is helpful to remind yourself that this is temporary and it won't be long until the cleanse is over. Below is a list of things you can do if it starts to feel like too much. We recommend starting at the first option and trying that for a day or two before moving on to the next option.

Protocols to let go of, in order of importance:
- ❖ Drop the Green Smoothie (page 86) and drink it when you can. Don't worry about doing it every day. Next time you are at the store or a local juice bar, pick up a vegetable juice or any green drink.
- ❖ Drop the Beet Tonic Salad (page 85) and do it when you can. Don't worry about doing it every day.
- ❖ Yoga
- ❖ Breathing
- ❖ Meditation
- ❖ Daily Self Massage (abhyanga)
- ❖ Exercise with Nasal Breathing

Here are some foods you can add:
- ❖ Add some snacks if you are feeling rundown, such as apples, sunflower seeds with raisins, pumpkin seeds with dried cranberries, or rice cakes with avocado and salt during the Pre and Post Cleanse.
- ❖ Add nonfat whey protein or lean meat if your blood sugar keeps crashing anytime during the Colorado Cleanse.

GENERAL FREQUENTLY ASKED QUESTIONS

Q: Does ginger have a different effect on us when it is simmering in water to become tea, or eaten raw (shredded/minced) and put for instance in a salad, or gently fried as in chinese mixed vegetables?

A: Ginger is called the universal spice because it balances all three doshas. It doesn't matter whether it is in a tea or eaten raw - it will have the same properties. Fresh ginger is preferred over powdered. I am not sure if the Chinese fried version will be as potent as fresh ginger.

Q: I see in your spring-list that you recommend eating dried fruits over fresh fruits. Why is that?

A: In the spring, everything is wet. The earth holds onto more water this time of year and so do we. Our mucus membranes are cleansing and we often see more mucus production. Thus all foods harvested in the spring are dry or at least more dry than summer and winter harvested foods. Fruits are eaten dry because in nature these fruits would not exist in a ripe form until summer. The only way to preserve them was to dry them. So they are acceptable in the spring. It is always better though to eat fresh, in season foods.

Q: My husband and I have been feeling hot in the evenings at dinnertime and after, especially flushed face feeling. Is this anything to do with the cleanse? I have some pitta imbalance, could it be due to that? Thanks for answering all of the cleansers questions.... you guys are great!

A: Yes this could be due to a pitta imbalance. As we enter the Main Cleanse this should even out. You may want to cut down on the hot water to help reduce pitta right away. It might be the beets - when you stop those this may help as well.

Q: Why don't we take the Warm Digest or Cool Digest before the ghee?

A: It is an option. But because we are resetting the digestive fire in the Post-Cleanse, I can let the digestive fire get somewhat lower during the Main Cleanse and the *Warm Digest* (or *Cool Digest*) isn't really needed. Traditionally taking *Warm Digest* (or *Cool Digest*) with the ghee is an option and not required.

Q: Each day after lunch I've gotten very gassy. For lunch, I've eaten salad greens, beets, sometimes avocado, rice crackers with sunflower seed butter, apple and apple juice. I thought it might be the apple juice and/or apple, but yesterday I omitted them and still felt a bit uncomfortable.

A: When we start such a high fiber diet this will begin to scrub the intestinal villi and can cause some digestive disturbance. When we start the Main Cleanse we will stop the high fiber diet and now start to heal the now cleansed intestinal villi. The gut should feel soothed by the kichadi diet.

Q: I know we drink a lot of lemon water on the post cleanse, what about Lemon water during the pre and main cleanse? I often have some lemon in my drinking water and first thing in the morning a glass of warm lemon water. Have not done it since the cleanse because you did not mention anything about it. Would like to know why not or if I can? How does lemon juice work?

A: Lemons will stimulate the digestive process and can be useful anytime. I don't like to drink only lemon water though as the rinsing effect of plain water is also valuable.

Q: Is one small bowel movement a day normal during the Main Cleanse?

A: Yes, this is perfectly normal. This is why we have you taking the *Warm Digest* or cool digest with the Main Cleanse. The metabolism is going to slow down and this is a normal process. If it becomes uncomfortable, then like I posted earlier - use an herb like *Trifala* or *Elim I* to keep things moving.

Q: I am gaining weight on this cleanse, and wondering what to do about that. I am doing most of my normal level of activity and training, though feeling really sluggish when training. Any advice?

A: Sometimes the body will not let the fat go until it is convinced the war is over. If life is very stressful, this may be a cause. The other cause could be slow digestion and you may need *Trifala* or *Elim I*. The other cause is that the blood sugar is unstable from grazing and is reluctant to burn fat. All this should balance as we finish the cleanse.

Q: Am I supposed to be losing weight as the fat burns? I am following protocol, but not necessarily shedding weight. How do I make sure I am burning fat to detox?
A: Weight loss is not the only determining factor if fat is lost. Weight is also affected by the lymph. If you're less hungry and not having a big appetite you are burning fat.

Q: Wow, I feel horrible today. I am just trying to understand if this feeling is from toxins being released or from not having enough food. Hard to know if it's blood sugar related or just those emotions being released. Is anyone else struggling? Are supposed to have these down days or if we are supposed to feel good the whole time? Thanks!
A: Up days are common and so are down days. These could be toxic release - if so drink more. They could be emotional release - if so it might help to practice random acts of kindness even though you have no desire to do so. You can also stop the herbs for a couple of days and eat more from Meal Options #2-4.

Q: My face has what looks and feels like a major allergic reaction. Is it a sign of detox?
A: It is hard to say - we are in allergy season and this may be a factor to consider. If you are really uncomfortable and sense that the cleanse is causing it, I would suggest to stop it for a couple of days and see if you improve. Restart the cleanse if there seems to be no effect. If you don't want to stop the whole cleanse, just stop the herbs and the water and see if that makes a difference.

Q: I was wondering if when the massage oil gets absorbed, does it interfere with fat metabolism? Or are the inside and outside oleation processes not connected at all?
A: The external oleation won't affect fat metabolism. The oil on the outside of the skin acts more as a carrier for the herbs in the oil to penetrate the cell wall. Much of the oil itself is too large of a molecule to penetrate the cell wall. External massage will oleate the intercellular tissue where the lymph drains waste, allowing for the drainage and removal of this waste to be more efficient.

Q: I'm finding that I'm retaining water in my legs and have a bit of edema. Is this normal? And what can I do to alleviate the situation?
A: This is a sign of some lymph sluggishness. Hot water and *Manjistha* can be increased. Take manjistha 3 caps, 3x/day and sip more hot water. Make sure you

are doing the self massage -- actually if you can do it toward your heart two times a day that would be good. Go back to 6 tsp of ghee and stay there until the end. Keep me posted. Perhaps a phone consult after the cleanse.

Q: What does it mean for those of us who are feeling sluggish and fatigued? What should we do to follow up on this?
A: Your body really hasn't jumped into the major fat burning stage yet, which means there is liver congestion and the digestive system is still stagnant. I recommend a consult so we can get to the bottom of it and fix it.

Q: My skin and mucous membranes are still feeling very dry from the low fat and nonfat diets, in spite of the all the morning ghee and all the water that I've been drinking.
A: This means there's a significant level of dehydration, which means your intestinal inner skin is dry as well. Read my video-newsletter about how inner skin determines what outer skin looks like at www.lifespa.com/skin.

We hope you feel lighter, calmer and inspired!

SUCCESS STORIES

I have not felt so clean and light in a very long time. **Since I have finished the cleanse my energy level has been amazing!**

I felt better through the whole cleanse. **I lost 10lbs** and felt lighter and cleaner. I had a lot of emotion that surfaced which I wanted to let go of too.

Wanting to stay true to the cleanse, I was able to resist snacking and notice how much of my munching was just mindless habit. I feel energized and light and am able to stick to 3 meals a day, no problem. **My husband was able to break his coffee/caffeine addiction.** He hasn't had any since the day before the pre-cleanse. He experienced no headaches and has no cravings!! We didn't do this for weight loss, but I **lost 6 and my husband lost 10 pounds.** A nice bonus as we head into the cold New England winter and heavier foods, holiday parties, etc. Both of us feel so good! We've both done many mini cleanses, and I've done 7-day panchakarma. This is by far the best experience we've had cleansing at home. Thank you!

The most dramatic improvement is that **my desire to snack is pretty much gone.** Specifically, the "habit" of grazing because I think I need food is gone. My energy is more stable throughout the day. I've lost 5 pounds. Skin is clearer. I love the self-massage oil!

I was experiencing Lyme disease like symptoms over the summer (big here in the east) with achy joints and fatigue. All that has gone away and my arthritic toe is starting to regain much of its range of motion.

I absolutely loved the cleanse. I've done a few cleanses/fasts in the past and the biggest difference this time around was the "no cravings." I also loved the daily emails of encouragement and reminders.

I lost 9 lbs. I feel good and calm. My skin glows, no wrinkles (and I'm 53). I'm in tune with the rhythm of the day. I'm sleeping great. No cravings. I'm a happy camper!!

Lost 6 pounds! Digestion feels easy and good again. I feel light and more grounded at the same time. I have also picked up some good habits that are easy to keep up.

I had done the four day cleanse and wanted to experience the colorado cleanse in hopes of boosting my digestive system, feeling less sluggish and tired. I did not know what to expect and so happy I did the cleanse. I lost about 5 pounds, fitting nicely in my size 6 now, I feel light, no longer wishing to eat heavy meals. I am preparing my meals and ensuring that they are in season and balanced. I was vegetarian and now enjoy a vegan diet. I feel great!!! I had my mom also on the cleanse..she was excited.. See you in the spring!!

I just love how I'm continuing to feel and look. I haven't been on a scale in years but know when I've lost or gained and I've shed some pounds especially in the last few days. Mostly I appreciate the calm energy I'm experiencing. My caffeine habit was minimal before (1 cup of black tea a day) but I can see now how very sensitive I am. Finding out how food affects my well being has shifted so much for me and I now feel I have some solid insights into how to create calm and stay feeling light...a delicious way to go through the day. Thank you!

My skin is clearer and more radiant, I lost 5 pounds and 5 inches from my body, my digestion feels great and more consistent, my chronic sinus induced sore throat is mostly gone, no cravings...

I had great success with the cleanse on a number of fronts. My mind and mood were calm and stable, **I cleared out resentments I was hanging on to from 2 old relationships,** I lost fat weight...from my thighs, belly, buttocks area and I feel clearer on the foods that I should eat for optimum energy going forward. All of these benefits are carrying through the end of the fast and are still true for me today.

This was my first cleanse and I thought the experience was very cool. I enjoyed eating the food on the pre- and post-cleanse and didn't struggle with the khichardi-only part of the cleanse. I am now still WANTing to eat a low-fat, mostly gluten- and dairy-free diet. I only lost a few pounds but am **feeling lighter and clearer**. Best of all **my long-term chronic problem with constipation is much improved**.

My energy is more even throughout the day, **I can't stop whistling** (starting to feel like one of the seven dwarfs), and I am **not as sensitive to environmental allergens**! This is one big reason I did the cleanse in the first place.

My **digestion has improved immensely** since I started the first cleanse, and it continues to get better even in the days after the fall cleanse. My digestion has been horrific for as long as I can remember, so this is a REALLY big deal! YAY!

I have **no word to describe how happy I am**. I lost 5 pounds. **I look unimaginably very good.** I am peaceful, different out look to life.

This was the first time I've done a cleanse like this so I didn't know what to expect. Although I got off to a rough start on the first day, it was smooth sailing after that. I was surprised how the cleanse carried me through a very busy and stressful time in my schedule and surprised at how quickly it went.

Along with weight, I feel I've **shed emotional baggage** that I've been carrying around for I don't know how long.

I feel really fantastic now that the cleanse is completed. My food **cravings have completely gone** away and I have no desire for cookies, coffee or sweets. I also don't feel like eating greasy egg dishes or cheese. This is quite a switch for me! I am very content with the seasonal fruits and veggies, especially apples. I also have experienced benefits from the yoga, meditation, skin brushing and oiling. I feel like my lymph system is running much more smoothly, and is not congested. I **lost about 9 pounds, and several skin problems cleared up**. I feel like the heat of the summer has calmed down in my body, and I am ready to enter the winter months full of clear and calm energy. Thanks for a fabulous experience!

Before this cleanse I was suffering from extreme perimenopause symptoms of anxiety at night. The first week I did experience some stress and had episodes of anxiety at night but they were not nearly as severe as they were before. By the beginning of week 2 the episodes diminished in severity about 70% and I was able to continue sleeping after each episode. Now in the post cleanse I have not had any episodes and although I still have hot flashes they are less in severity also. ...I have no desire to ever do another "crash diet" again - not after knowing how good it feels to feel good. My thinking is clearer and I feel more balanced. I am excited about how great I will feel as I continue with this program and regain my good health. Thank you!!

This cleanse was even better than the first. I felt stronger, more focused and comfortable during this cleanse. I was able to eat (3) solid meals each day with no snacks and my appetite decreased significantly. I definitely went into fat burning mode and got rid of not only food toxins but emotional ones as well. It was **cathartic and very enlightening**. Thank you Dr. Douillard for your support and guidance throught out the cleanse.

...the **spots on my hands got lighter**.

Hi, I **lost 9 pounds** and feel much better because of it. I feel lighter and somewhat more energized. I've done both cleanses and they've been very helpful.

Lost 4 to 5 pounds and have kept it off.

I have **given up my addiction to diet Dr Pepper** and as small as that sounds I no longer have that jittery energy. I am getting connected to my body:)

I've had a fatty deposit in my upper thigh for a few years. I feel that it has reduced in size during the cleanse!

Lost about 10 pounds. Felt very calm and balanced during the main cleanse. **It has been easy to continue with a healthy diet post-cleanse.**

The cleanse worked like clockwork for me. **I lost 8 pounds beginning to end and am so far keeping it off**. I believe I have reset my metabolism and my digestion and have had no compunction to dive back into indulgent eating habits.

The set up and structure of the cleanse and the support system left no room for unanswered questions or confusion. All the materials were thorough, professional and very clear. I look forward to the spring cleanse, hopefully with my husband and maybe some friends!

Thanks again you wonderful Lifespa people! The cleanse- my second with you- was again a life changing experience. **I am now within 5 pounds of my high school graduation weight and I am 56 years old! I had learned that I have celiacs disease about 5 months before the last cleanse. I had changed my diet but just wasn't seeing results. I truly felt so awful all the time I wasn't sure how much longer I could go on. I was also about 25 pounds over my preferred weight and feeling so sluggish and bloated. The cleanse was just what I needed to undo all those years of poisoning myself! Between changing my diet and repairing my digestive system, I feel like I am living in a different body!** I just assumed that aches and pains were a part of being fifty-ish! This summer I took in all of my pants and after this second cleanse I think I can go down a second pant size!

I expected that my RA symptoms would benefit from the cleanse and they did, but I also experienced fewer seasonal allergy symptoms.

I am sleeping great since the cleanse. Prior I would wake up at 1 or 2 AM and not fall asleep again until 4ish. Also my **mood is more consistent** not so many ups and downs. **Very few hot flashes.**

I **lost about 8 pounds** during the cleanse and I feel lighter and calmer.

I am obese and over 3 years ago, I started on a journey to shed my excess weight. After dropping about 60 pounds, I became stuck on a plateau and despite all of my efforts (whole food diet, cardio, strength training, calorie counting, etc.) I could not budge off of the plateau and as a result, the yo-yo dieting started again and I wound up regaining some of the weight I lost. This went on for nearly 2 years (seriously) until I did the Spring 2010 Colorado Cleanse. I lost 15 pounds during the cleanse and have been losing weight steadily ever since! I lost 10 lb. during the Fall Cleanse and as of now, **I have lost about 60 pounds total since the May cleanse**. I understand the cleanse isn't about losing weight but I truly believe that detoxing my fat cells and cleaning and healing my GI tract has truly fundamentally changed how my body works. I am thrilled!

Every time I do the short home cleanse or the Colorado Cleanse it gets easier and easier. This time around I have had **amazing energy** even though I was battling a cold going into this. It has really helped me think about why and when I eat. I am more determined than ever to stay the course and continue eating my 3 meals a day and eating with the seasons. I don't want this great feeling to end! :)

Before the cleanse I had been feeling sluggish and tired quite often. Starting with the main cleanse, I began to **get my energy back**. Also, I had been having problems with my digestion, feeling bloated and gassy. That went away during the cleanse.

I **lost 7 pounds** and feel much lighter overall, **less bloated around the abdomen than before**.

I definitely feel better and received compliments on my 'glow.'

Four weeks after the cleanse I am able to easily stick to three meals a day with no more mid afternoon sugar crash and cravings!

Since I finished the cleanse my cravings and snacking have been eliminated. I eat two to three healthy meals and feel satisfied with **even energy** throughout the day.

The most apparent change I've experienced has been a **consistent good night's sleep**. I'm highly stressed as a caregiver, and sleep is my most precious commodity. **I'm very grateful**.

I felt so well supported by the eBook, daily emails, conference calls, and emails with friends hundreds of miles away who were also doing the cleanse, that I never needed the support of the LifeSpa staff.

Excellent, informative, instructive. I love the added dimension of the calls and also that the ayurvedic herbs help the body help itself and not become dependent on them.

I really enjoyed the camaraderie, even though I'm a thousand miles away. I felt supported in my effort, which gave me the initiative to stick to it!

I really like the personal/daily support. I appreciate how knowledgeable/accessible Dr. John is; **the cleanse is like a two week hands on/experiential workshop.**

I really enjoyed the e-book, daily e-mails and the great response time from the Life Spa staff. Although I could cleanse again on my own with what I've learned, it **felt so much better to do it with others.**

I have never been involved in a structured cleanse before with outside assistance. I personally didn't send questions but **reading answers to other people's questions was extremely helpful.**

After having to deal with weird health issues that no one could explain to me for more than a decade (especially doctors), this has been the one thing that has worked best for me. Am I back at 100%? Not yet. But even if I did not have the opportunity to improve my health with future cleanses, I feel so much better now that I'd be OK feeling as good as I do now for the rest of my life. But, why stop now? :0)

This was a great experience and I hope to Colorado Cleanse twice a year for many years to come. This was a very effective 21st century application of ancient Ayurvedic wisdom.

This isn't an easy cleanse but man, the **effects are completely worth the effort**. I have several friends that have cleansed with me. **One has actually eliminated her food sensitivities, mild asthma, skin rashes and congestion. How amazing!**

It's amazing how great you feel.

I was happy to be able to eat all the way through, so I could be with my family at meals, even though I ate different things. Also it was a great experience to be satisfied with much less food than I was used to expecting to need to eat. It still is!

I have already mentioned it to several friends and acquaintances. They don't want to wait until Spring for the next one!

Again nice price. Great support. So much better than any trendy cleanses out there.

I find Dr. Douillard very well-educated and articulate. I appreciated all the background and explanation for the reasons we were doing certain parts of the cleanse. I find him very credible and professional with a lovely manner.

Having done the master cleanse - I see the difference in a starvation cleanse and this one.

Yes, I recommended it to my husband this last time and we both enjoyed going through the process together, **ending the cleanse with Panchakarma was the best!**

As an editor for such publications as Yoga Journal and Natural Health, I see a lot of "detox plans." Most are based on good intentions and pseudoscience. I enrolled in the Colorado Cleanse because I knew from first-hand experience — multiple interviews — that John Douillard was the real deal. This is a cleanse based on a clear understanding of body dynamics. It's not about suffering — fasting, denial — but about working with your own body rhythms to create better health. My own results were undeniable. **I lost 11 pounds. More important, my blood pressure dropped from 160/98 to 125/75. That is a HUGE gain in health.** Thank you, Dr. Douillard. *~Kind regards, Hillari Dowdle*

I cannot believe how good I feel having done this cleanse. **My energy and spirits feel so healthy and my sense of well being has been restored.** Thank you. I have followed many restrictive diets and eating programs before. However, having the information and support of Dr. John put me in a place of truly feeling as if I was doing exactly what my body needed. It was a good feeling.

During the [Colorado Cleanse] pre cleanse, my digestive system changed so dramatically. The speed of the change really surprised me. ... **Digestive pain gone, bloat almost gone and I lost eight pounds by day six of the cleanse. Amazing, I only lost weight from my middle.** Additionally, I've struggled with cystic acne for several years; By the fourth day on the cleanse, my skin looked incredibly different. **Existing cysts are healing, no new cysts and the texture of my skin improved dramatically.** Let me tell you, I've released more than toxins.

The Colorado cleanse was life changing for me in many ways. I have been ill for about 8 months. Without this painful experience, I wouldn't have discovered how Ayurveda can benefit my family and realized how much the digestive system plays an enormous role in our wellbeing. ...I had multiple hospital visits, doctor visits, tests after tests leading nowhere. I started the cleanse and... **a miracle.** I started feeling this inner calm that was amazing, my body wasn't fighting anymore. It seemed to be at peace. **My anxiety has faded away and my energy is back.**

I wanted to express you my gratitude for what you have shared with us during the cleanse. During the cleanse I had several things to do like: cook every day for my family (I have 2 kids), bake a cake for a community pic-nic and go out for dinner with friends... and, hard to believe at least for me, I was so happy with my Khichadi that I didn't mind at all to have around other kind of food! It was amazing! I really enjoyed every single day of the cleanse. My little one, almost 3, said when she grows up, she will do the "detok" with me! Thanks again!

Great Cleanse, wonderfully explained, well done research and transmitting of the very important information and knowledge, **made me understand things I tried to get for years.** It makes so much sense!!!

I lost 9 pounds!

This is the best cleanse I have done. The pre cleanse was key. I felt fantastic going into the main cleanse and so it was so much easier. The post cleanse was also very helpful. I LOVE the daily emails - really kept me on track. **I am not craving the usual stuff, my ovarian cists are gone, energy is good and my mind is clear.** I am looking forward to the next one!

Knee pain almost gone, lost weight, feel better, digestion good thus far (and it has not functioned well as long as I can remember!!!)

More energy and more of a feeling of lightness in my body.

I can overcome the desire for food, treats, wine, etc. because I have come to understand the temporary nature of this cleanse. There will be more cake, wine, more Starbucks in my future if I so choose. That is another powerful concept...if I so choose. So what if we apply this to other things in our lives? What would happen if we approached a problem with the understanding that it is temporary? Would that challenge be easier to navigate (as has become the case for me with this cleanse)? Would we make different choices? Would we just let things happen to us? Or would we CHOOSE. We have free will. What do you choose for your life? Manifest!

I feel great. **I have no cravings for sweets.** I actually have started telling myself a story that I am allergic to sweets.

The swelling on my legs is completely gone.

I dropped about 8 pounds-yes! I do feel lighter and more healthy.

My chronic indigestion is improved. I do feel I've moved towards a healthier me. I've felt a bit calmer as well.

I'm feeling more in tune with my body. Yesterday I felt great, finally feeling the positive effects. Clear and energized. **I also felt it helped me face some emotional eating issues I had stored.** So thank-you so much. Great job everyone.

My skin is smoother. I lost 12 pounds which was unexpected!! I am going to continue with the diet as it really suits me. I have tried to lose these 12 pounds for many many years!!! Caring about the food I am eating.

Wow! I lost 10 pounds that previously would not budge. I was amazed at my lack of hunger and general disinterest in foods outside of the cleanse regimen, yet I was never at a loss for energy. **I've received many comments that my skin looks great (I'm a longtime acne sufferer).**

I liked that the whole staff was doing the cleanse with us. It helped to know Dr. John was bummed about not eating cake and how he overcame that desire. :)

The ease of which it could be adapted to my day. I have an insanely stressful job, yet I made it through at level 1 for all protocols. I love having all the educational insights provided in the calls, email & website. Thank you! And I love that the effects of the cleanse keep on going.

This is an amazingly powerful and thorough cleanse that doesn't disrupt your life. I also found the daily emails and forum helpful to create a sense of community and let me know that others were experiencing similar feelings or reactions along the way. Thanks for developing this! My body is calmer and happier with three meals. Thank you!

Thank you for taking the time to follow the
Colorado Cleanse and take care of your health.

We are grateful to share this important information with you.

We hope the Colorado Cleanse has inspired you to
make more positive changes in your life.

May you be happy, health, and strong!

ALSO AVAILABLE AT LIFESPA

Receive Dr. Douillard's Free Bimonthly Health Reports

Dr. Douillard sends free Health Reports and Videos 1-3 times per month with the latest research, health tips, and exclusive discounts.

- ❖ Reports on how to be healthy and happy
- ❖ Powerful wellness education
- ❖ The latest nutritional research
- ❖ Special discounts

Recent Health Reports:

- ❖ Stop a Cold in its Tracks
- ❖ Memory, Mood and Focus Super Herb!
- ❖ Never Take This Vitamin
- ❖ Boost Immunity Now!
- ❖ Prevent Diabesity - The Next Epidemic
- ❖ Researchers Rediscover Longevity Herb
- ❖ Treat the Cause of Insomnia
- ❖ Avoid Dangerous Herbs
- ❖ Staggering Reduction in Cholesterol and Inflammation
- ❖ Don't Be Fooled By Your Sunscreen
- ❖ Look and Feel Vibrant in 3 Steps
- ❖ Home Sinus Therapies That Prevent Colds and Allergies
- ❖ The Miracle of Lymph
- ❖ Love Unconditionally on the Road Less Travelled
- ❖ Top 10 Proven Weight Loss Tips
- ❖ Lose Stubborn Weight Effortlessly
- ❖ Turn Stress into Joy in One Minute
- ❖ Vitamin B12: Almost Half of Americans are Deficient!
- ❖ Iodine Deficiency Linked to Cancer and Disease

Sign Up Now at www.lifespa.com/news!

Guided Colorado Cleanse
Each Spring and Fall

Detox Retreat at Home with:
- ❖ Live Conference Calls with Dr. Douillard
- ❖ Daily Emails that Guide, Inspire and Educate
- ❖ A Community of Fellow Cleansers

Would a Guided Cleanse Be Better For You?
Is it hard for you to cleanse by yourself?
Do you feel overwhelmed or isolated?
Do you want to have the best cleansing experience possible?
Do you want to learn as much as possible

What is the 'Guided' Colorado Cleanse?
Each spring and fall Dr. Douillard guides a group of cleansers through the Colorado Cleanse with live conference calls, daily emails and our online forum. Join our community of hundreds of fellow Colorado Cleansers around the country – and the world – and share recipes, encouragement, ideas and support with new friends committed to better health.

We announce the dates in our free Health Reports.
Sign up at www.lifespa.com/news.

The Colorado Cleanse Supply Kit Has Everything You Need
Anytime of the year you can purchase the Colorado Cleanse Supply Kit, which includes all of the supplies you need for the Colorado Cleanse at a bulk discount: all herbs (*Turmeric Plus, Liver Repair, Manjistha, Regenerate, Warm Digest* or *Cool Digest, Beet Cleanse,* and *Sugar Destroyer*), a week's supply of khichadi, ghee, castor oil, and lymphatic massage oil. During the Guided Colorado Cleanse each spring and fall it is offered at a deeper discount.

Learn More
www.lifespa.com/coloradocleanse

Also by Dr. John Douillard

Books
Body, Mind and Sport
The Mind-Body Guide to Lifelong Health, Fitness, and Your Personal Best

Perfect Health for Kids
10 Ayurvedic Health Secrets Every Parent Must Know

The 3-Season Diet
Eat the Way Nature Intended: Lose Weight, Beat Food Cravings, Get Fit

The Encyclopedia of Ayurvedic Massage

The Yoga Body Diet
Slim and Sexy in 4 Weeks Without the Stress

DVDs
Ayurveda for Detox
Ayurveda for Stress Relief
Ayurveda for Weight Loss

Audio CDs and MP3s
Ayurveda for a Healthy Family
Ayurvedic Skin Care
Enjoy Exercise with Ayurveda
Heal Anxiety & Depression
Lose Weight with Ayurveda
Restore Energy with Ayurveda
Sleep Better with Ayurveda
The Miracle of Lymph
Ayurvedic Pulse-Reading Course

Available at www.lifespa.com

Services at LifeSpa

Dr. John Douillard's LifeSpa
6662 Gunpark Dr E, Suite 102
Boulder, CO 80301
(303) 516 – 4848 or (866) 227 - 9843
www.lifespa.com | info@lifespa.com

LifeSpa's Mission

After studying alternative medicine for the past 30 years with leading experts from around the world, it became clear to me that, while the body is infinitely complex, the best medicine is incredibly simple.

It is my mission to help us transition from a culture of expensive and complex health care to a culture that seeks optimal health through natural mind-body medicine, leaving us more self-sufficient, rather than dependant on a medical system or a pill. ~ *Dr. John Douillard*

Ayurvedic Consultations with Dr. Douillard

www.lifespa.com/consults

Dr. Douillard is available for private consultations in person or over the phone. Through a comprehensive exam aimed at uncovering the cause of what ails you, Dr. Douillard diagnoses and treats the fundamental imbalance that may be responsible for all of your symptoms. Therapies may include, but are not limited to: herbs, diet, exercise, lifestyle changes, and stress prevention.

Chiropractic with Dr. Douillard

www.lifespa.com/chiro

Dr. Douillard has provided chiropractic treatment to Olympic and professional athletes including Billie Jean King, Martina Navratilova and the New Jersey Nets Basketball team. Dr. Douillard uses techniques similar to Active Release Technique, which is a state of the art soft tissue technique that provides rapid and lasting results. He spends at least 25 minutes with each patient, and 80-90 percent of that time is working on the soft tissue. His goal is to achieve 50-80 percent improvement in the first visit. In most cases the condition is resolved in 3-5 visits, depending on how many years the condition has existed.

Panchakarma Rejuvenative Detox Retreats

www.lifespa.com/panchakarma.

Panchakarma is a series of detoxifying, balancing, and nourishing therapies performed over a series of 3, 5, 7 or more days. Panchakarma is not just a detox program. This is only its side benefit. It is a Transformation in consciousness - replacing stress with silence. During your Panchakarma you will receive Ayurvedic spa treatments every day with one or two therapists. You will also meet with Dr. Douillard regularly to unravel old emotions, beliefs, habits, and patterns that contribute to the stress which is typically the under-lying cause of most disease. Each day during your free time you will enjoy a customized practice of rejuvenative yoga postures, breathing techniques, meditation and self-inquiry, along with a special cleansing diet and herbal support. We will send you home with a maintenance plan of herbs, yoga routines, dietary recommendations and stress relief techniques all tailored to your unique needs and goals.

Therapeutic Ayurvedic Spa Treatments

For Relaxation and Rejuvenation

If you live in the Boulder/Denver area or are passing through Colorado, enjoy a 1- or 2-hour Ayurvedic Spa treatment with our loving and skilled Panchakarma therapists. We can design the perfect treatment for you based on your goals, such as detox, sinus decongestion, relaxing muscles, or calming the mind. To book your treatment, simply call our office at 303.516.4848 and let us know what your goals are and we will design the perfect treatment for you!

Self Help Herb Store

www.lifespa.com

LifeSpa offers only the highest quality herbs, nutritional supplements and products to support you on your journey towards optimal health. Our interactive website helps you understand which herbs or supplements will be best for you.

All Natural Ayurvedic Skin Care
A Revolutionary Preservative-Free and Chemical-Free Product Line
www.lifespa.com/skincare
Products that are loaded with preservatives and chemicals are perceived as foreign to the body. This perception by the body triggers an automatic rejection of these products and they are not able to penetrate deep into the tissues. Lifespa skin care products contain no preservative or chemicals. Because of this, the body recognizes Lifespa products as nourishment guaranteeing the deepest possible penetration. At LifeSpa we believe that what you put *on* your body is as important as what you put *in* your body. The Skin Care Line includes *Hydrating Mist, Facial Moisturizer, Wrinkle Serum, Cleanser/Toner, Facial Mask* and *Body Butter*.

What is Your Ayurvedic Body Type and Skin Type?
www.lifespa.com/healthquiz
Take one of our free interactive questionnaire to learn how you can stay balanced and healthy with the best foods, herbs and lifestyle practices for your body type.

Speaking Engagements with Dr. Douillard
Dr. Douillard is available to lead workshops, seminars, conferences and lectures. Please contact LifeSpa for more information.

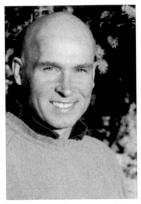

John Douillard, DC, PhD is the former Director of Player Development for the New Jersey Nets and has written and produced 18 health and fitness books, CD's and DVD's. Dr. Douillard publishes a nationally known bi-monthly video-newsletter on current health issues and cutting edge nutritional research that you can sign up for at www.LifeSpa.com. He just released his latest book, *The Yoga Body Diet* and is the author of *The 3-Season Diet; Body, Mind, and Sport; Perfect Health for Kids* and *The Encyclopedia of Ayurvedic Massage.* He is the creator of the LifeSpa Ayurvedic Skincare and Herbal Line and currently directs LifeSpa, an Ayurvedic Retreat Center, where he offers consultations (in person or over the phone) and personalized Panchakarma Detox Retreats. He lives with his wife and six children in Boulder, CO.

Dr. John Douillard's LifeSpa
6662 Gunpark Dr E, Suite 102
Boulder, CO 80301
(303) 516 – 4848 or (866) 227 - 9843
www.lifespa.com | info@lifespa.com